LESSONS IN LEADERSHIP

The importance of leadership in public services has increased dramatically in the past five years as politicians around the world have sought modernisation and reform.

The authors of *Lessons in Leadership* argue that leadership is not mystical and mysterious. They look at how ideas of visionary leadership have been developed and discuss their applicability to the public sector. Case study material from around the world is used to illustrate some of the issues around leadership and the role of politics. This book also provides a detailed analysis of an organisation that seemed beyond help. The authors offer an assessment of its characteristics as a learning organisation, its journey to developing leadership capacity and ambition.

Readers of *Lessons in Leadership* will have a greater understanding of:

- various theoretical perspectives on leadership
- the tensions that can arise between the bureaucratic, administration-driven traditions of public services and the leadership and management styles required within new and emerging operating environments
- the relationship between political leadership and organisational leadership
- different approaches adopted by public service leaders around the globe, including generalisable attributes of success and failure
- which existing theories of leadership are appropriate for a new public management context or whether new models or paradigms may be required to move forward

Lessons in Leadership will be invaluable reading for students of public administration, particularly those on MBA and DMS courses, as well as practitioners and policy makers in the public services.

Eileen Milner is Programme Director, Information and Knowledge Management, London Metropolitan University.

Paul Joyce is Head of the Department of Strategic Management and Marketing in the Nottingham Business School, The Nottingham Trent University.

Eileen Milner dedicates this book to Richard D. C. Atkinson.

LESSONS IN LEADERSHIP

Meeting the Challenges of Public Services Management

Eileen Milner and Paul Joyce

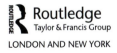
Routledge
Taylor & Francis Group

LONDON AND NEW YORK

First published 2005
by Routledge
2 Park Square, Milton Park, Abingdon, Oxon, OX14 4RN

Simultaneously published in the USA and Canada
by Routledge
29 West 35th Street, New York, NY 10001

Routledge is an imprint of the Taylor & Francis Group

Typeset in Baskerville MT 10.5pt by
J&L Composition, Filey, North Yorkshire
Printed and bound in Great Britain by
TJ International Ltd, Padstow, Cornwall

British Library Cataloguing in Publication Data
A catalogue record for this book is available from the British Library

Library of Congress Cataloguing in Publication Data
A catalog record for this book has been requested

ISBN 0-415-31905-6 (hbk)
ISBN 0-415-31906-4 (pbk)

CONTENTS

FOREWORD

The purpose of this book is to study how managerial leaders can be successful in the public services. While there are some excellent books that deal with one or more aspects of leadership, none has quite catered for our interest in researching prescriptions for managerial leadership in the context of modernisation and public sector reform. Howard Elcock's *Political Leadership* is a recent contribution but its scope is quite wide-ranging, including studies of politicians as well as managers and considering not only classical theories but also contemporary debates about local government political structures. Heifetz and Linsky's book *Management on the Line* is very good on the role conflicts and personal aspects of leadership but takes a general look at leadership and adaptive change. Philip Heymann's *The Politics of Public Management* and Mark Moore's *Creating Public Value* are both excellent books, which have certainly influenced our own book. While both of these are very concerned with strategy and strategic management in the public sector, they come closest to what we have attempted to do in our study of leadership.

We have been attempting to identify how successful managerial leaders see things, what their values and beliefs are, what they pay attention to, and what they do when they bring about modernisation and reform. We have relied very heavily on case studies, although we have also examined published research.

In this book we want to offer the reader our understanding of the lessons for people taking on the responsibility of leadership in the public services. Of course, such lessons as we outline here are based on events that occurred in specific situations and involved specific sets of people. Anyone reading these lessons faces two challenges in learning from these lessons. First, there is the challenge of reconciling the lessons with their own pre-existing network of beliefs and values. Some of these lessons might not be easy to absorb and may sit uneasily with other beliefs and values that have proved their value to the individual over a long period of time. Secondly, the circumstances in which the lessons are to be applied might be subtly or substantially different from those occurring in the case studies. This would mean the lessons might be applied selectively or only after judicious modification. Despite these difficulties, our case studies and our outline of lessons in how to be a successful leader offer the reader three opportunities:

1. to use these case studies to supplement their own direct observations of leadership problems and processes,
2. to compare their reflections on successful leadership with our lessons in leadership, and
3. to identify ideas suggested by our lessons that could be the basis of their own practical experiments in leadership behaviour.

OUTLINE OF THE REST OF THE BOOK

In the chapters that follow we will be on the hunt for clues about the reality of leaders and the consequences they have for public services improvement. We will be looking at how success is achieved by leaders. Is it all down to their ability to find a vision for the future of their organisations? Do they look into the future to make sure the vision is one that can be achieved? Are they, as popular management theory would have us believe, brilliant at being in touch with the people in their organisation? Are they exceptionally gifted communicators who can put a vision across in a way that inspires? Are they inspiring the people who work in their organisations to innovate and provide a better service to the public? We will see that there is evidence to support the idea that leaders are making a difference to the reform of public services.

We can say now that what you will read will not show that leaders are superhuman, although they are quite special and dedicated. The evidence will show that successful leaders are people with admirable personal qualities. We will see that they are people who have managed to help their organisations adapt to changing times and thereby reconstruct an improved relationship to the needs of the society we have today.

In Chapter 1 we will look at leadership and reform of the public services and highlight the political and democratic context of this leadership of reform. In Chapter 2 we will be presenting the results of our survey of the academic research literature. One of the main benefits of this survey is a more detailed look at the idea of visionary leadership and its applicability to the public sector. In Chapters 3 and 4 we begin to draw on case study material from around the world to understand in more detail some of the issues around leadership generally and the role of politics in particular. One point we make is that successful public service leaders are not just the same as leaders in other sectors. We are also keen to make the point that the reform agenda is more than reorganisation, because it involves adaptation and/or renewal.

In Chapter 5 we have a go at defining leadership for the public services. We suggest that it is not mystical and mysterious. We also use case study material on Brisbane City Council in Australia to look at leadership. The key themes are broadly in line with the view of leadership that we label an enabler perspective (see Chapter 1).

Chapter 6 contains three upbeat case studies, each of them showing how a public services leader was able to bring about adaptation of their organisation. This chapter acknowledges the role of political support, leading through vision, and communicating and persuading staff. However, the cases also show how the critical contribution of the managerial leadership depended on the specific situation. This chapter also underlines the need for successful leaders to be resilient and able to cope with personal attacks.

Chapter 7 is a detailed analysis of the experiences of a council in the north of England. It involves an assessment of its characteristics as a learning organisation and in particular how it developed leadership capacity and ambition. This chapter is concerned with renewal and not just adaptation, by which we mean the development of a capacity for continuous adjustment and adaptation.

Chapter 8 is our final chapter and we draw together all the lessons in leadership emerging from the preceding chapters. It becomes clear that the evidence on leadership we have collected for this book places us in the position of viewing leaders as people who enable change and renewal. These are the strong themes of the experiences analysed – the leaders are not elitist or playing merely ideological games. They are leaders who serve by enabling the public services to catch up with cultural changes in modern societies and they do this by helping their organisations to learn, albeit this is sometimes a painful and uncertain learning process.

CHAPTER 1

LEADERSHIP AND REFORM OF THE PUBLIC SERVICES

INTRODUCTION

Our contribution to the study of leadership in the public services in this book is based on the idea that public service leaders help to create and realise possibilities for 21st century organisational learning and adaptation. The need for leaders at the beginning of the 21st century is, in our opinion, in large part a result of the problems created by the way the public sector has lagged behind developments in society. The public services now have to catch up. This is not easy. The public services are in truth struggling to match cultural changes and life-style trends that had begun manifesting themselves in the 1960s and 1970s. In the process of adapting the public services, the managerial leader has not only to help their organisation change but also personally to learn how to manage their interdependence with elected politicians and apply political skills in the process of managing performance and change.

There have always been innovators in the public services, but the pressure to reform and modernise the public services is predominantly political. We begin, therefore, by emphasising that people have been turning to leadership in recent years because there has been a political drive for the reform of public services. This has been supported in the UK by investments in leadership development in health, local government, police services, education, and elsewhere in the public sector.

The message that leaders matter in the public services has also been reinforced by the creation of awards to recognise individuals that have shown leadership in the public services. In Britain, during 2004, David Henshaw was recognised for his achievements as a leader when he was awarded a Public Servants of the Year Award (see Chapter 7). In 2001 the winner of this same award for leadership was Andrew Geddes, who had been an Inland Revenue director. In 2002 the winner was a fire fighter, Danielle Cotton, and in 2003 the winner was Ian Hobson, a head teacher. In the last case, Ian was credited with transforming the school he led:

> 'Hobson used his leadership skills to transform a school that was in danger of closure when he became head in 1998 . . . he has inspired staff and colleagues to perform at a higher level.'
>
> (*Public Finance*, 3–9 October 2003: 21)

In this book we will be examining the leadership experiences of public services managers and we will be emphasising the lessons of this experience. There is evidence from our case studies suggesting that in democratic societies leaders are capable of bringing about big improvements in the interests of the public. However, we will not be emphasising a single universal experience of leadership. For we have found that what individual leaders actually do depends upon the nature of the situation they find themselves in and the actions of others in the situation, especially elected politicians. In the best sense of the word, leaders have to act pragmatically in the circumstances they face.

In this first chapter we begin by noting the emergence of leadership as a public policy issue. Then we explore some of the overarching perspectives taken on leadership. We see this as important for the reason that some arguments and confusions about leadership are not so much disagreements about the advantages and disadvantages of this or that type of leadership as disagreements about fundamentally different perspectives on leadership. Consequently, by recognising these perspectives we can isolate arguments about choice of ways of seeing leadership from arguments about the theoretical causes and effects of leadership action. This chapter then explores the notion of leadership by managers of public services in a democratic society, which we begin by considering the Weberian view that the democratic politician is at a disadvantage in relation to the bureaucratic expert. Finally, we take a look at the claim that at the beginning of the 21st century the welfare state societies created over the preceding 100 years to provide more security to individuals and families are subject not only to severe strains but also to attempts to reconstruct them into new welfare states. By the end of this chapter we hope we will have established key features of political and social history that are very important to an understanding of the present and future possibilities of leadership in the public services.

IS THERE A LEADERSHIP PROBLEM IN THE PUBLIC SERVICES?

A recent UK government report by the Department for Education and Skills and the Department of Trade and Industry (2002: 3) observed:

> 'We are conscious that good leadership is as vital to the success of the public sector as it is elsewhere in the economy. We are committed to much better delivery of our public services. This cannot happen without significant improvements in the quality of public sector managers and leaders and those in the voluntary and social enterprise sectors.'

The situation in the public sector services was seen as, if anything, even worse than that in the private sector. The Department for Education and Skills and the Department of Trade and Industry (2002: 11) commented on a survey by the Chartered Management Institute:

> 'A Chartered Management Institute report (2001) suggested that half of all junior managers rated the quality of leadership in their organisations as poor. Disappointingly, the public sector leadership received the lowest ratings.'

These official expressions of concern were just one indication of the increased recognition of the importance of top management in the public services. There was also other evidence, albeit anecdotal. This included reports of Chief Executives of poorly performing public services organisations losing their jobs, and the growing use of consultancy firms to headhunt for executive talent.

In the case of the UK's public services, one reason for the growing interest in leadership was concern about the capacity for change and innovation in public services organisations. Sir Michael Bichard made this point succinctly in the Foreword to a study of public sector leaders:

> 'In most organisations leadership is the key which unlocks or blocks change. The public service is no different, so the consistently poorer ratings accorded to public sector leaders is a key cause for concern during a period of major reform.'
>
> (Charlesworth *et al.* 2003)

At the outset of the 21st century the UK government went further than merely talking about the importance of leadership and began investing in leadership development. It set up bodies for developing leadership in all major sections of the public services, including health, local government, the civil service, schools, further education, and the armed services. For example, the National College for School

Leadership was set up in November 2000; the NHS Leadership Centre was established in early 2001; and the defence services set up a Defence Leadership Centre in April 2002. In the case of the health services the linkage to the reform agenda of modernisation was very evident.

We should underline here that in Britain people were saying the issue was not just one of management generally. A distinction has been drawn repeatedly between management and leadership. It has been suggested that whereas managers plan and exercise control, leaders inspire and motivate followers. This claim for the effects of leadership comes through to some extent in the quote above about Ian Hobson, who it is suggested had inspired his staff to perform at a higher level and had transformed his school. Many influential and thoughtful observers of developments in the public services have also recently emphasised the need for leadership that is visionary, which seems a plausible proposition if we are hoping to see public services managers and workers who have been inspired by their leaders. Some see such visionary leadership not merely as capable of improving organisational performance but also as capable of producing organisational transformation. Michael Bichard, a successful public servant and it has been said an inspirational leader himself, not only distinguished leadership from management but also linked leadership to transformation when he wrote:

> 'In the recent past we have spent a lot of time and rhetoric on improving public sector management and nowhere near as much on leadership. Yet it is leadership that we need in this new millennium, because it is leadership and not good management that transforms organisations.'
>
> (Bichard 2000: 44)

PERSPECTIVES ON LEADERSHIP

Leadership, it might be said, is a universal feature of human civilisations. Kellerman and Webster (2001: 510) claimed that leaders 'are in our nature' and suggested we are 'hard wired to, in one or the other role, engage in the leader–follower dynamic'.

Some of the varying reactions to the word leadership no doubt stem from understanding the leader–follower dynamic in different ways. More than 70 years ago one thoughtful observer of management reflected on the wisdom of using the word 'leader' because of what it conveyed. In a paper presented at a conference in 1928 Mary Follett (1941: 291) said:

> 'I have sometimes wondered whether it would be better to give up the word "leader," since to so many it suggests merely the leader–follower relation. But it is far too good a word to abandon . . .'

The issue that concerned Follett was the danger of a view of a leader as someone who gives orders to followers who are loyally obedient and carry out the orders. This meant that the leader was the author of the end result and followers mere tools for the execution of the will of the leader.

The issue of the leader–follower dynamic did not disappear when in the 1980s the study of leadership headed off into a new direction and became interested in the way that leaders were responsible for strategic missions and visions and for their communication and sharing (Bass 1985; Bennis and Nanus 1985). One of the popular new theories concerned what the academic world has called transformational leadership. Among others, Bass (1985) suggested that transformational leaders obtain a level of employee performance that exceeds expectations. This idea of transformational leadership is normally defined in opposition to transactional leadership.

> 'Whereas transactional leadership is described as a series of exchanges between leaders and followers, transformational leadership goes beyond exchanging inducements for desired performance by developing, intellectually stimulating, and inspiring followers to transcend their own self-interests for a higher collective purpose.'
>
> (Boehnke *et al.* 2003: 5)

Academics point to the need for transformational leadership behaviour such as visioning, intellectual stimulation, team building, coaching, and inspiring. For example, the leader creates 'intellectual stimulation' by the provision of new ideas and causing people to rethink ways of doing things.

The new theories have been considered relevant to public service settings. This may be possible where the theory is kept at a very general level of abstraction. Thus it is suggested that typically leaders inspire and motivate others to transform the performance of an organisation. Commonly, it is explained how this occurs through communication and role modelling, and how, as a result, employees are empowered and take some responsibility for the performance and success of the organisation (Duncan *et al.* 1995).

A belief in the need for leadership, especially for strong leadership, whether it is political or managerial, makes some people uneasy. In the distant past there was sometimes uneasiness because of egalitarian and democratic values, and hopes for increased fraternity. H. G. Wells, a Fabian socialist, apparently once said that in the past people relied on great leaders – Buddha, Mohammed, etc. (Follett 1941). In democratic societies, all individuals should count and there should be scepticism about reliance on great leaders. But the role of leadership in the public services of a modern democratic society needs to be debated and examined. There is no necessary implication that leadership is bad for democracy. Arguably, leadership is compatible with all manner of social relationships, from authoritarian to democratic ones. We pick up this discussion of democracy and leadership again later in this chapter. In more recent times the uneasiness has been at times associated with a left-wing critique of various forms of discourse as being implicated in power relations, which we will discuss shortly.

We want to offer here an outline of three main perspectives on leadership, which for convenience we have labelled the elite perspective, the discourse perspective, and the enabler perspective.

An elite perspective is a framework of beliefs and assumptions that regard leadership as a process whereby leaders of public service organisations have the answers to the big strategic questions and they then communicate them to followers. The source of the answers may be seen as the leaders' intuitions or their superior intellect or their access to clever advisers. But irrespective of the source, the leader is assumed to know best and is assumed to communicate to managers and employees a vision for where the organisation is going. Moreover, while the implication is often that the leader is not interested in exercising detailed control over others but enjoys substantial influence, the elite perspective may gloss over problems in exercising influence and the operational limits of this influence.

Traces of this elite perspective can be found in the descriptions of British trade union and political history. For example, in the late 1880s trade union membership rapidly spread among dock workers and other unskilled workers on the back of successful industrial action led by Tom Mann, John Burns, and Ben Tillett. The leaders of this 'new unionism' were said to be more highly skilled workers inspired by socialist ideas and comprised of individuals who wanted to see trade union organisation spread beyond the ranks of skilled workers. They included orators who held up a vision of a better way of living to the unskilled workers:

> 'When Burns spoke upon Tower Hill to his dockers only a small part of his speeches were devoted to Union demands: a large section was turned to urging them to behave as human beings – not to beat their wives, not to fight one another savagely, not to drink themselves stupid at the first opportunity. The most oppressed and unhappiest of human beings, those who were nearest to the animal, now had recovered their humanity and demanded their rights. They took as their leaders those who were most fiercely in opposition to respectable society . . .'
>
> (Cole and Postgate 1949: 426)

In some ways we could compare this example of external socialist leadership of the union organisation of unskilled workers, with the argument made by Lenin in the early 1900s that a political (social-democratic) consciousness had to be brought to workers because by themselves they could only develop trade union consciousness. He argued that the role of the political party was to educate the working class and develop its political consciousness. He portrayed the party as the leadership of the working class, bringing to it a political consciousness that it lacked. Again we can see an elite perspective on leadership, in which the leaders have the ideas and the answers and the followers have to learn from the leaders.

In turn we can present a very different kind of British socialist movement from a century ago that aspired to have an elitist influence in society and shape public services as well as other aspects of national life. Fabian socialists were compassionate intellectuals who believed that reform and improvement could be based on expert knowledge (MacKenzie and Mackenzie 1977). Sidney Webb, a key figure in the circles of Fabian socialists, argued in 1901 for a brains trust for national revival and in 1902 assembled a group of experts to work out how national life could be made more efficient. The group was called the 'Co-Efficients'.

'In the congenial company of the Co-Efficients Sidney was associating with men who believed, as he did, in the cult of the specialist, who wanted strong leadership, who favoured large efficient units, whether these were great powers, big commercial enterprises or agencies of public administration. Above all, they were avowed elitists, intolerant of the cumbersome and apparently wasteful processes of democracy, who wanted to see England ruled by a superior caste which matched an enlightened sense of duty with a competence to govern effectively.'

(ibid.: 291)

The motivation of the leader is not essential to the definition of elite leadership. The individuals concerned may have good intentions and work tirelessly to improve the situation of ordinary people. But, by definition, they are experts who apply their special insight and expertise, say, to solve social problems and to mobilise the organisational capacity of the public services on behalf of the public.

A very different perspective on leadership was offered by a section of academics in the 1980s and 1990s. They viewed leadership not primarily as behaviour but as a concept within a 'discourse' on the management of the public services. We would guess that Foucault, who looked at historical documents to understand how definitions of illness, criminality, and sexuality developed, was probably an inspiration for this type of attention to management discourse. When applied to leadership and management, Foucault's work suggests we look at management discourse as being based on technical knowledge but also see that this discourse has power over other people. In fact, some academics began referring to the adoption of private sector management discourses within public services organisations and described it as, in effect, an ideological process that impacted on power relationships within the public services. Newman and Clarke (1994: 13), for example, put this rather forthrightly as follows:

'We want to argue that the place of management in the transformation of public services needs to be seen as arising from a more complex set of relationships . . . we need to understand that management is more than a technical specification of functions or skills, it is also a social group with a particular ideology (managerialism) through which it lays claim to both social and organizational power.'

(Newman and Clarke 1994: 13)

The academics argued that this private sector management discourse displaced the previous discourse of public administration and policy implementation. In fact, it was also argued that there was more than one variant of the discourse. The specific content of one discourse might be seen as neo-Taylorism since it focused on control to achieve efficiency and productivity, while another was a 'new managerialism' that emphasised the leadership role of managers in inspiring employees to meet the needs of service users and to innovate (Pollitt 1993).

It can be argued that these discourses are 'purely ideological' in the sense of rhetorical claims for the power of managers to be recognised and accepted; however, Newman and Clarke (1994) expressed the view that the discourse of new managerialism (which defined managers as leaders) was of increasing practical significance in the late 1980s. Either way – as a rhetorical claim or as an ideology with practical significance – the discourse of new managerialism was considered to be favourable to the power of managers. They suggest (1994: 25) that bureau-professionals were being turned into managed and managers as a result of being subjected to the two discourses; they said:

'these managerialisms aim to construct identities in and through relations of power and practice.'

(Newman and Clarke 1994: 25)

Managers gained power, as they became leaders who directed the public services and defined the public as customers or consumers rather than citizens. The writers in this perspective may also have assumed that the main losers in terms of power are, or will be, elected politicians and public service professionals. There is a flavour of this perspective in the following suggestion by Clarke, Cochrane and McLaughlin:

'Put crudely, reference to "customers" may simply allow managers the freedom to make a rhetorical claim to have their interests at heart in their conflicts with the staff whom they manage, without the actual position of the "customers" necessarily being improved. Redefining those for whom welfare organizations are responsible as "customers" may make it easier to manage staff from above.'

(Clarke et al. 1994: 6)

According to this quote, the discourse of new managerialism is an ideology that gives power to managers over professional and other staff but does not have to produce benefits for the public. Clarke and his colleagues did, however, consider it possible that the public might also be winners from this management discourse, gaining influence and access to opportunities and resources.

What can be said about the underlying attitude of this discourse perspective in respect of the value of management and managerial leadership? Just as Foucault was interested in resistance to the power of specialist groups to define others, writers on the public services who analysed management discourse might also end up explicitly or implicitly concerned with the existence and extent of resistance to the encroaching power of management. For example, Newman and Clarke touch on resistance briefly in the following way:

'The depth of resistance to change among those in bureau-professional regimes has a number of dimensions, not all of which are encompassed by Conservative explanations of their unwillingness to surrender power.'
(Newman and Clarke 1994: 26)

But we must be careful not to oversimplify the views of those taking this perspective. It is possible to work largely within a discourse perspective and yet to see that resistance is not the only issue. Newman and Clarke, for example, appear *not* to be nostalgic for the days of the old welfare state when politicians relied on professionals to define public needs and decide on how services should be organised and delivered:

'It was not only the neo-conservatives who were critical of the paternalism of state welfare, its concentration of political and professional power, its limited conceptions of the needs of service recipients, its intrusive and oppressive bureaucratic processing of people as cases.'
(Newman and Clarke 1994: 26)

This discourse perspective represents an improvement on the elite perspective in at least one particular – it emphasises the conflictual potential of issues of power and ideology in leadership processes that the elite perspective glosses over. Its big weakness, however, for those interested in the modernisation of the public services and democracy is that the discourse perspective provides little or no basis for developing a theory of leadership *for* the public services. This is because it is so preoccupied with proclaiming the loss of power by professional employees and politicians that it (largely) ignores the responsibility of those running public services in a democracy to adapt them to match the public's changing needs and, therefore, for continuing to reconstruct on a better basis the relationship between the public and its services. In addition, and more obviously, it is so interested in drawing attention to discourse that it is in danger of ignoring the practice of leadership.

The enabler perspective of leadership, certainly as expressed through the work of Heifetz and Linsky (2002), not only recognises the conflictual aspects of leadership processes and emphasises the practice of leadership, it also recovers some of the positive spirit of the elitist perspective but without the elitism. Its first key proposition is that there is a dangerous aspect of leadership that arises when answers cannot be supplied from the people at the top and there is a necessity for learning to take place. Heifetz and Linsky (2002: 13) emphasise the presence of uncertainty about what to do and a lack of knowledge in their following statement on the challenging nature of learning to adapt:

> 'Leadership would be a safe undertaking if your organizations and communities only faced problems for which they already knew the solutions . . . But there is a whole host of problems that are not amenable to authoritative expertise or standard operating procedures. They cannot be solved by someone who provides answers from on high. We call these adaptive challenges because they require experiments, new discoveries, and adjustments from numerous places in the organization or community. Without learning new ways – changing attitudes, values, and behaviours – people cannot make the adaptive leap necessary to thrive in the new environment.'
>
> (Heifetz and Linsky 2002: 13)

The anti-elitist view of leadership articulated here is partly revealed in their judgement that there are problems that 'cannot be solved by someone who provides answers from on high'. In a situation where there are no obvious answers, the leader has the task of encouraging experimentation and discovery.

A second key proposition is that leaders facilitate learning and adaptation by their organisations. Part of the way that leaders facilitate learning and adaptation may be through vision statements. Where leaders are seen as using a strategic vision to create a sense of direction for moving from the present to a desired future of the public service it is not necessary to see this vision as originating with the leader in a personal sense. Instead leaders who enable strategic changes may find or construct a vision by listening to people in the organisation, asking questions and being receptive to ideas already in existence (Bennis and Nanus 1985). There can be a creative aspect to this:

> 'If there is a spark of genius in the leadership function at all, it must be . . . a kind of magic, to assemble – out of all the variety of images, signals, forecasts and alternatives – a clearly articulated vision of the future that is at once simple, easily understood, clearly desirable, and energizing.'
>
> (Bennis and Nanus 1985: 103)

Bennis and Nanus also stress the unusual personal capacity for learning they believe to be characteristic of leaders. 'Leaders are perpetual learners' (Bennis and Nanus 1985: 188). But because many leaders are also key to the occurrence of effective organisational learning, there is the possibility that the implementation of change can be brought about through non-coercive methods. They specifically envisage this organisational learning as involving the challenging of conventional assumptions and the deepening understanding of the organisation's role in its environment.

The third key proposition of the enabler perspective is that there are often opponents as well as allies and people in the middle, and the leader has to handle all of these groups in enabling the organisation to adapt. The leader has natural allies who share the vision, opponents who have a lot to lose by changes, and some who may resist change simply because change is disruptive. The enabler perspective is not naïve about, or blind to, conflict. 'Leadership, then, requires not only reverence for the pains of change and recognition of the manifestations of danger, but also the skill to respond' (Heifetz and Linsky 2002: 48). So, learning and adaptation is not always safe and not always comfortable for those concerned – there is uncertainty in the situation, conflicts in the organisation, and dangers for leaders, as well as plain inertia. One of the key implications of this account of the enabler perspective is that leaders need to be skilful in a process that can be conflictual and requires both experimental and improvised behaviour by them.

These three perspectives clearly present radically different ways of looking at leadership. It may not always be clear immediately to which of these three (or some other) a researcher or commentator on public services leadership adheres. It is also obvious, in our opinion, that there is something to be gained by reflecting on these perspectives even if there are reservations about them. For example, the discourse perspective, with its critical evaluation of the management/leadership discourse that has entered the public services in recent years does at least provoke questions about the motives of managers in using this discourse. Is the discourse a self-serving ideology aimed at enhancing their power, or will public service users also see benefits as a result of the application of leadership? The enabler perspective is helpful, we would argue, in identifying the experimental nature of strategic change and thus the risks and dangers of leadership – is it therefore reasonable to see leaders as having a monopoly of power, or is their position vulnerable too if the experiments fail? We intend in writing this book to work mainly in line with the enabler perspective, and from here on largely assume that way of looking at things.

MANAGERS OF PUBLIC SERVICES IN A DEMOCRACY

We have been looking at some very different ways of framing leadership and now we think it is important to set leadership in the public services in its political context. We do this by highlighting some issues about the political aspects of managerial leadership in the public services.

The first issue concerns the relative power of top managers in the public services and the elected politicians. Max Weber provided a very pessimistic account of the relationship between democracy and bureaucracy, a view that is bound to be depressing for anyone who holds democracy to be one of the most important achievements of modern society. This view was an element in his diagnosis of the advance of bureaucracy in the early decades of the 20th century. We think he was putting forward two key propositions. First, while the officials who managed the administration of the state were required to carry out formally and rationally defined roles, they were nevertheless experts in relation to the politicians. Secondly, because they were experts this meant that the elected politicians who were nominally in control were not in fact able to control the officials, and in that sense democracy was subordinated to bureaucracy. Weber summed this up as follows:

> 'Under normal conditions, the power position of a fully developed bureaucracy is always overpowering. The "political master" finds himself in the position of the "dilettante" who stands opposite the "expert," facing the trained official who stands within the management of administration.'
>
> (Weber 1970: 232)

American public sector scholars have challenged this Weberian view in recent years (Heymann 1987; Moore 1995). Based on case studies of the work of top public service leaders, they concluded that achievement of strategic goals depended not only on organisational capacity but also on the support of the elected politicians for strategic plans to achieve the strategic goals. As Moore (1995: 22–3) expresses it, managers in the public sector are involved in 'managing upward, toward politics, to invest their purposes with legitimacy and support'. While the elected politicians lack the detailed knowledge of the problems and needs being met by a public service organisation and they lack the detailed knowledge of the organisation itself, which makes them dependent on the appointed managerial leaders, the managerial leaders depend on the politicians for various things, including legitimacy and financial resources.

Another key idea in the relationship of elected politicians and government officials is that of the party-political neutrality of the latter. This seems to be an obvious requirement for any system of representative democracy based on regular elections and party competition for political power through elections. An implicit assumption is that representative democracy can carry the full burden of ensuring that elected politicians understand the priorities and wishes of the public. During an election the political parties make promises to the public and get elected on their manifesto. The guarantee of the representativeness of the government is that they were victorious in the elections. Since the government therefore knows what the public requires, it passes laws and makes policy decisions and the civil servants should simply and loyally implement policies to the best of their professional abilities. If there is a change of electoral fortunes for the party of government and a rival party takes over the responsibility of government, then it is assumed that the public has a new set of priorities and wishes, and the civil servants are expected to loyally implement the policies of the new government. This is made easier if the civil servants adopt an official attitude of party-political neutrality. Consequently, their job is to give advice to elected politicians on how new policies might be best adopted and do their best to implement political decisions effectively, but they must not become supporters or partisan.

Of course, the democratic world is more complex than this. In the UK, for example, there is a relatively small number of advisers appointed to support the elected officials who are given ministerial responsibilities in government. These advisers are in appointed posts but they are expected to be political, supplying advice and ideas on what might be done. Yet again in some countries there have been experiments with the use of fixed-term contracts for some of the top civil servants. Then there are also some systems of government (e.g. federal government in the United States) where incoming governments appoint large numbers of officials, and these same officials can be replaced in huge numbers when the government changes. A comparison of the UK and US systems suggests that there is a trade-off as far as the civil servants are concerned: permanence and job security are given in return for party-political neutrality, and if civil servants are politically partisan then they cannot expect to have job security.

It has been argued, however, that the tradition of impartiality no longer makes sense in a world that is more complex and more dynamic and governments are no longer confident of statist solutions to societal problems. It is not so much that officials should now become highly party-political as that the culture of professional impartiality and distance that created a lack of responsibility for policy success now seems questionable. Since a statist posture by the government seems less tenable, the government needs to work with other stakeholders to define the nature of the problems and to identify possible solutions. In other words, what was assumed to have taken place through the electoral process of representative democracy now takes place partially through problem-solving at various levels, and which may involve officials as well as elected politicians. So, in a specific sense the officials have taken on a political role, although it is not precisely the same as a party-political role.

One of the pressures on politicians that brought this about is the increasing political difficulty about the level of taxation and the exact use of the revenue from taxation. In the early 1950s the proportion of ordinary people in the UK paying income tax was relatively small, and the amount they paid was small. By the mid-1970s the ordinary family was losing a large part of their income to taxation, and political parties promising to bear down on public spending in order to reduce income tax became popular. The Labour Party only became electable in the 1990s when it was no longer seen as likely to increase income tax. One consequence of this is that politicians become more hesitant about seeing the obvious solution to societal problems as being a public sector response requiring funding out of taxation. If there are other ways of solving problems, working with other stakeholders in the problems, these alternatives are at least worth considering. But even if a traditional approach is adopted to problem-solving, requiring a government programme and public spending, then politicians should want to make sure that the expertise of the officials is used to ensure that public money is well targeted.

This sounds like a very complex situation for a managerial leader in the public services to handle. No one is officially asking them to become politically partisan, but they are expected to be more active in the search for solutions to societal problems and more active in steering government programmes and interventions to the correct target. They are, in other words, to remain politically neutral while being more political. They are less able to hide behind the convention that says 'politicians tell us what to do and we simply implement their decisions'. The politicians may want their judgement on what hitherto would have been regarded as a political decision about priorities in terms of needs and problems. The politicians may also want them to meet with and secure a consensus with external stakeholders on what is to be done. This means managerial leaders learning how to manage the dialectic of sometimes 'taking a stand' and sometimes being prepared to take on board the views of others. Moore puts this point very well:

> 'In political management one cannot entirely rid oneself of the pleasure and obligation of having and articulating a point of view; nor can one rid oneself of the obligation to learn and integrate the views of others. It is through such dialogue that the best chance of finding and successfully pursuing public value probably lies; it is this potential that should be cultivated by the techniques of political management.'
>
> (Moore 1995: 149–50)

REMAKING THE WELFARE STATE

We think it is essential to a proper understanding of the current nature and possibilities of leadership in the public sector to note the pressures for reform on social-democratic political cultures and the welfare state models found in Western Europe and elsewhere. In the second half of the 20th century, in Britain and other countries, a social-democratic culture was dominant in the design and delivery of public services. This culture represented a strongly statist view of the way to improve the lives of the average citizen. The old welfare state of the 20th century has many fine achievements to its name. It provided higher levels of security as well as health, welfare and education services to large numbers of people. For over 25 years the economy was managed to provide full employment. And all these achievements, in Britain in any case, were not just achieved by the 'public sphere' in general, but by the state in particular.

But it had its defects too. These defects did not seem so very important in the early days. They stemmed in part from what is variously referred to as both 'modernism' and 'paternalism'. Essentially, citizens could hope for an improvement in their lives but all that they were required to do was vote in general elections for political parties that promised to establish and maintain the welfare state, pay taxes, and grant the power to act to the state itself. Since the public ceded the power to act, the state could act only through the employment of professionals and experts. In the absence of public involvement, these public sector professionals designed the welfare state services and were depended upon by the state to properly understand the needs and circumstances of ordinary citizens and the kinds of services they needed. When this failed to be the case, the welfare state was being bureaucratic. The welfare state suffered from one of the deficiencies of (old-style) modernist states – it thought it knew and it imposed standard solutions that did not quite fit the needs of individuals.

The welfare state in Britain, with both its achievements and defects, survived in the 1950s and 1960s reasonably well, but its statist defects showed up in the 1970s, and were followed by political consequences in the 1980s and 1990s. In common with many other countries the welfare state expenditures came to be seen as a burden and people began to discuss the fiscal crisis of the state. Initially, it seemed that the difficulties were going to be resolved by the election of right-wing governments that would return society to a pre-welfare state based on the ideas of liberal capitalism. In fact, in the 1990s it became apparent that British society was finding it difficult to afford the welfare state and the kind of dependency culture and disincentives to work it was alleged to create, but that it was not prepared to ditch the welfare state either. And paradoxically because, under the Conservative Government, unemployment rose steeply, the consequent costs of unemployment benefit were rising too. It was therefore difficult to keep public expenditure down. Other problems emerged for the Conservatives in reducing the size of the welfare state. For example, however disappointed the public was with the British National Health Service, this did not mean that it was ready to abolish it. This posed an enormous governmental dilemma: the welfare state is both essential and has political allegiance and at the same time is a major economic and political problem. Politically, for so long as the Labour Party went into elections with pledges to increase taxation they lost the elections. It was only when they made it clear that they would not raise income tax that they won two clear mandates in 1997 and 2001.

In Britain, the response to the dilemma of the welfare state has been to embark on the modernisation of public services and to create a new welfare state. Whilst governments with two very different ideologies and very large majorities have been doing this for 20 years, in truth, this work has barely begun. It is not an easy political strategy and it is not yet clear that it can be delivered. This is the set of conditions in which leadership in the public services is now operating.

Leaders became seen as key to this reform agenda. They were required, to quote Bennis and Nanus (1985), who were speaking more generally, to change things by 'creating dangerously'. It is a pity, but this idea of leaders creating dangerously has not received much attention, although the linking of leadership and danger was thoroughly explored later by Heifetz and Linsky (2002). One obvious aspect of reform that creates danger is that change may fail and the leader may be blamed for the failure. The manager who leads experiments in public services reform and fails can expect to be criticised by politicians and the media for wasting public money and taking chances. Moore (1995) warns that failures will be noticed and attacked by the media and politicians. 'Against such a background, public managers can withstand some failed experiments, but they cannot endure a long succession of them' (Moore 1995: 233). This means that leaders in the public services have to manage political risks of failure as well as the usual risks of change failing.

CONCLUSIONS

The underlying assumption of this book is that, despite individual differences, leaders in the public services generally share a commitment to improving the public services, making them more up-to-date, more effective, and more efficient. They are, in other words, through their actions trying to make the public services better. However well the public services are managed and delivered, leaders want to see them get better. This makes them agents of change and innovation. This is consistent with current definitions of leaders as people that create or strive to create change (Kellerman and Webster 2001).

In this chapter we have argued that leadership in the public services is seen as a matter of great significance for the future of the welfare state. We would sum this up by saying that politicians are seeing leaders as the change agents who will radically reconstruct services to form a new welfare state and thereby replace the traditional modernist model of welfare state services that made the public clients. The new welfare state seeks to end the client status of the public and put them first. This involves renegotiating the status of public services professionals and the constraints on making change and improvements. This poses challenges and difficulties to leaders that should not be underestimated.

CHAPTER 2

WHAT CAN WE LEARN FROM ACADEMIC RESEARCH?

INTRODUCTION

A key proposition in Chapter 1 was that public sector management was not enough for the new millennium, and that leadership was needed because public services organisations had to be transformed. This is a political judgement. It involves taking a practical point of view. But what are the facts on this matter? To consider this properly, we need to consider the possible existence of various forms of leadership (e.g. charismatic leadership, visionary leadership) that exist, analyse the processes of leadership (how it works), analyse the results of leadership, and so on. This is the aim of this chapter. The studies that have been selected are mostly very recent and are based on samples that either are entirely public sector or include a substantial number of people in the sample who were public sector managers. We also offer a normative model of public services leadership based on a recent large-scale survey. This chapter should be useful to sensitise the reader to the key concepts of leadership as we examine a number of case studies in the chapters that follow.

We have one point to make before we turn to the academic research on leadership. From the very early days of studying leadership in industry it has been possible to approach the concept of leadership in different ways. First, there has been the tendency to assume someone is a leader by virtue of a formal position. Thus a Chief Executive may be regarded as the organisation's leader simply because she or he is the Chief Executive. Secondly, leadership may be conceptualised as a set of practices and the person doing them as a leader. Accordingly, it might be argued that a leader is someone that analyses situations and then mobilises the organisation through decisions, advice, encouragement, and recognition. Thirdly, yet another tendency is to see leadership as an expression of personal qualities. For example, people are leaders, it might be said, because they are exceptionally strong, brave, and resolute. Our point is that we are not convinced it is wise to restrict studies of leaders to any one of these three tendencies. It may be argued that all three refer to things – position, practices, and personal qualities – that are interwoven in varying and complex ways. We need to be sensitive to the possibility of this interweaving.

We have tried to be critical in our reading of the academic research on leadership in the public services, but in actual fact this has proved difficult because the quantity of such research is still limited. We are seeking through this review of empirical studies to become clearer about the processes of leadership and the relationships leaders have with significant others.

LEADERSHIP AND MANAGEMENT

Kotter (2001) appears to have had a tremendous impact on people who write about leadership, including those who write about the public services. Kotter outlined the nature of leadership in a series of binary oppositions between leadership and his definition of management. He said managers bring order and consistency. Leaders help organisations cope with change. Managers plan and budget. Leaders set a direction for change. Managers control by monitoring against the plan and then solve the problems revealed by the monitoring. Leaders motivate and inspire. Managers organise people; leaders align people. Managers design organisations; leaders communicate to people in a way that aligns them to the direction the organisation is going.

His style of presenting these binary oppositions is persuasive. He even carries this through to an overall diagnosis of the business world when he writes (2001: 85): 'Most U.S. corporations today are over-managed and underled. They need to develop their capacity to exercise leadership.' Others, also influential, have said much the same thing.

However seductive the view offered by Kotter, his work of distinguishing leadership and management is largely a definitional exercise. It is not difficult to come up with other definitions that cut across his definitions. For example, Kotter uses the word 'planning' in a very particular way and his definition of management has its roots in the 1970s rather than the 21st century. Some strategic planning models that were developed in the 1980s and 1990s for the public services prescribe the use of strategic planning as a process that can absorb both strategic issues and visions of desired future states. Moreover, strategic issue management can be a creative form of strategic problem-solving. So a planning process and problem-solving, which Kotter associates with management, are integrated with creative change in line with a vision of a future state, which Kotter links to leadership.

On the surface there is an immediate problem for us in that he defines leadership and management, we guess, principally with large

US corporations in mind and there is little in these definitions that takes account of the different stakeholders and relationships in the case of public services leaders. For example, there is no reference to elected politicians, who are important in the case of public services. On the plus side, his explication of these definitions provides many useful ideas that are to be found in other writing and research. For example, he stresses how leaders align people through communications. Secondly, he endorses the idea of empowerment through leadership communications. Thus he believes that the communication of the vision and direction enables lower-level employees to act and use their initiative. Thirdly, he underlines the importance of leadership credibility. He (2001: 90) writes: 'Many things contribute to credibility: the track record of the person delivering the message, the content of the message itself, the communicator's reputation for integrity and trustworthiness, and the consistency between words and deeds.' We pick up this point about credibility below, when we look at leaders and followers.

Bennis and Nanus (1985) carried out a North American study of individual leaders that provided them with conclusions that correlate very closely with the main themes of leaders and leadership outlined by Kotter. Their data were obtained from 60 private sector Chief Executives and 30 public sector leaders. They initially looked for similarities among the group but could not immediately find any obvious explanation for leadership success. Nor did they establish any different patterns for the private and public sectors. Continued persistence with the analysis eventually paid off and they produced a model to describe a pattern of behaviour that typified the leaders.

They emphasised how leaders were interested in results and how they sought to focus the attention of the people in their organisations through a strategic vision. Fairly conventionally, the strategic vision was seen as a mental image of a desirable future state of the organisation, and as key to creating a sense of purpose and direction. They wrote (Bennis and Nanus 1985: 90): 'With a vision, the leader provides the all-important bridge from the present to the future of the organization.' For them, there was an issue about the vision being owned by the people in the organisation. Leaders, therefore, have to communicate and get people behind the organisation's goals. So the leader must assemble the vision but then it 'has to be articulated clearly and frequently in a variety of ways' (ibid.: 143). They do have notions of empowerment and alignment, and see these as resulting from the successful sharing of the vision:

'This empowers individuals and confers status upon them because they can see themselves as part of a worthwhile enterprise. They gain a sense of importance, as they are transformed from robots blindly following instructions to human beings engaged in a creative and purposeful venture . . . Under these conditions, the human energies of the organization are aligned towards a common end, a major precondition for success has been satisfied.'

(Bennis and Nanus 1985: 90–1)

Then the next aspect of the process of leadership is using the vision to position the organisation. The leader first takes action to position the organisation and then works at sustaining the position. This, according to Bennis and Nanus, is important for the growth of trust in leadership.

The final important aspects of leadership concern capacity for development, both a personal and an organisational capacity. Their conclusions on this may be summarised as follows. Leaders have a capacity for personal learning. Leaders know their strengths and their weaknesses and they know how these correlate with the needs of the organisation. Leaders are good at learning, and good at improving their skills – they are self-evolvers. Some leaders, but not all, are also good at getting their organisations to learn. Indeed Bennis and Nanus conclude that it is leadership that explains why some organisations are good at innovative learning.

> 'We said that most of our ninety leaders were very much aware of the impor-
> tance of their own learning abilities and needs ... Fewer of them were
> equally conscious of their roles in organizational learning, but we did find evi-
> dence to suggest that much of their behavior served to direct and energize
> innovative learning.'
>
> (Bennis and Nanus 1995: 203–4)

Leaders stimulated learning by serving as role models and by rewarding learning when it happened.

These, then, essentially, were the main conclusions of Bennis and Nanus. Leaders assemble a vision, communicate it, share it, unify people in the organisation behind it in a sense of common purpose, and use it to position the organisation. In addition, they provide role models for individual learning and some of them direct and energize innovative learning by the organisation. Finally, Bennis and Nanus made some fleeting references to the idea that leaders align the energies of managers and employees. For example, they stated: 'Under these conditions, the human energies of the organisation are aligned toward a common end, a major precondition for success has been satisfied' (Bennis and Nanus 1985: 28). This idea about leaders and energy for change processes was later repeated in the private sector studies of strategic change by Pettigrew and Whipp (1993).

As we noted in Chapter 1, according to Bennis and Nanus, leaders do not act as some intellectual elite in the sense of bringing answers to the organisation. While Bennis and Nanus did conclude that leaders used judgement as well as creativity to formulate the vision, they also stated that leaders have also to be good at listening and asking questions because the vision is not down to them alone and needs to have some resonance in their organisation.

The study by Bennis and Nanus was not intended by them to test hypotheses and certainly it was not intended to test the ideas of Kotter. They reported that their method of analysis was inductive. They discovered their conclusions within the data and (as we noted) at first had found it difficult to detect a pattern. As we said above, the conclusions do seem to broadly fit Kotter's conceptualisation of leadership and to have little in common with Kotter's ideas of management. We conclude, therefore, that Kotter's ideas have some basis in reality.

TRANSFORMATIONAL CHANGE

Despite all the interest in transformational change, the only study we have reviewed that is a straightforward study of transformational change is a North American case study by Frost-Kumpf et al. (1993). They collected data on a successful transformational strategy at Ohio Department of Mental Health, between spring 1983 and late 1986, a period of less than 4 years. In what sense was it a transformational change? In this period the department changed its mission and goals, its services, its methods of service delivery, its operating structure, and its allocation of resources.

This transformational change was analysed as strategic change. The researchers identified and analysed more than 120 strategic actions. These actions were classified into a smaller number of action themes: gaining external support, building internal capacity, developing technical expertise, utilising training, taking symbolic actions, developing new programme thrusts, empowering key constituencies, developing alternative sources of revenue, responding to opposition, and co-aligning streams of strategic action.

The list of action themes is interesting. The first and second items on the list – gaining external support and building internal capacity – put us in mind of Heymann's (1987) model of strategic management in the public sector, which emphasises the way a strategic plan is intended to develop external support and organisational capacity to achieve a strategic vision that relates to social need. Of more immediate interest is the reference to symbolic action as a theme. This is because Frost-Kumpf et al. explained that it was top management that was taking symbolic action.

The symbolic actions included speeches and the publication of documents. These actions were a signal from the top management that the department was to be transformed. They expressed a strategic vision of a future in which the department played an entirely new role in meeting the needs of people with mental health problems.

'These actions communicated new concepts and values while emphasizing the possibilities for action and effective change in the future. The director's language expressed a new vision about what Ohio's mental health system could become and marked an irreversible break with past policies, service philosophies, and operating procedures . . . the director gave momentum to the change process . . .'

(Frost-Kumpf et al. 1993: 143)

So, we have confirmation yet again that vision plays a vital part in change, supporting the earlier conclusions of Bennis and Nanus (1985) and many others who have written about leadership. But we also have support from this analysis for the idea of transformation through empowerment. People were affected by the ideas and language of leaders. They acted upon the new concepts and values.

> 'The strategic language of the director nullified past issues, prior operating philosophies, and traditional practices in the department while giving form and substance to a new strategic direction. Through such language, numerous opportunities were opened for new ideas, actions, policies and programs. The importance of this particular language cannot be overstated.'
>
> (Frost-Kumpf *et al.* 1993: 151)

This is, perhaps, the best evidence we have that visionary leaders who communicate new ideas and new futures can encourage action by people in their organisations and that this can be very important to the realisation of transformational change.

LEADERS AND FOLLOWERS

As we have seen in a preceding section, leadership is often defined as different from (and complementary to) management. We have touched on the ideas of the role of leaders in communicating and sharing the vision with followers, and then empowering them to bring about a common purpose. In some cases, discussions of visionary leadership fade into discussions of charismatic leadership. It will be seen that little evidence on the importance of charisma yet exists in respect of public services leaders. We will be counter-posing the concept of leadership credibility to that of charisma. Then we look at a number of studies providing evidence on the effects of leaders on led. We will finally look at possible factors supporting visionary leadership. These factors include strategic decision-making, rewards, and culture management.

Charisma

Despite the popularity of the concept of charisma, we should note the lack of evidence about the importance of leadership charisma as an explanation for the readiness of public services employees to take up the leader's vision. Max Weber's writing on charismatic authority, often used as a starting-point, suggested that this type of authority was 'resting on devotion to the specific and exceptional sanctity, heroism or exemplary character of an individual person, and of the normative patterns or order revealed or ordained by him' (Weber 1947: 328). He also intruded a relational dimension into his account of charisma (Bryman 1992), which can be seen in the following quote. He wrote:

'In its pure form charismatic authority has a character specifically foreign to everyday routine structures. The social relationships directly involved are strictly personal, based on the validity and practice of charismatic personal qualities.'

(Weber 1947: 363–4)

We might make two suggestions about the meaning of this quote. First, charismatic leaders are not followed because followers have developed a set of routine responses or habits that comprise being loyal and obedient. They follow because they see something special in the personal qualities of the leader. We might imagine the led reacting to a leader by saying: 'I follow you and your vision because of the person you are, not because you are an incumbent of a specific position.' But secondly, perhaps the quote also means that the social relationship between the charismatic leader and the led is unstable. Perhaps his reference to the 'validity and practice of charismatic personal qualities' implies that followers want proof of the charisma of the leader (see Bryman 1992: 25). Consequently, perhaps followers withdraw their consent to be led when leaders no longer demonstrate that they have these personal qualities?

There has been a recent study of charismatic leadership in the public sector by North American researchers but its findings did not provide convincing evidence of the effects of charismatic leadership nor, in our opinion, did it use a proper operational measure of charismatic leadership (Javidan and Waldman 2003).

Javidan and Waldman began by interviewing several middle-level public sector managers about desired or prototypical leadership attributes in senior management. They then used these interview findings to construct items and they tested them with another 20 middle-level managers using a definition of charismatic leadership that the researchers had produced. They formulated a hypothesis about charismatic leadership characteristics that is summarised in Table 2.1.

Table 2.1 Javidan and Waldman's Charismatic Leadership Hypothesis.

Behaviour	Qualities
Vision articulation	Self-confidence
Optimism and enthusiasm	Eloquence in communication
Encouragement	High energy or endurance
Risk-taking	Desire for change

Source: Javidan and Waldman (2003).

Their next step was to produce a 37-item questionnaire that they gave to 203 subordinates of 51 upper-middle and senior managers from government organisations and asked them to judge the managers' behaviour and qualities. They also asked the managers' immediate bosses to judge the results or effects of each manager.

The study did find some evidence that the managers affected the self-esteem of their staff. If subordinates judged these managers as encouraging them to take responsibility and to think independently, as providing feedback and recognising good performance, then the self-esteem of the manager's staff was judged to be higher by the managers' bosses. Also if the subordinates perceived the leader as willing to accept risks to his or her status, power and promotion in order to achieve the vision, then, again, the self-esteem of the staff was judged to be higher by the managers' bosses. But none of the measures of charismatic leadership that Javidan and Waldman constructed was associated with perceived loyalty to the manager or the perceived relative performance of the manager's unit compared to the performance of other units reporting to the same boss. These results caused Javidan and Waldman to question the consequences of charismatic leadership in the public sector. They concluded that charismatic leadership might not provide performance or motivational results in the public sector in the way that it produced them in private businesses.

Trust and credibility

It may be recalled that we noted above that Bennis and Nanus discussed the existence of trust in the leader and connected this to the persistence of the leader in positioning the organisation in line with the strategic vision. Presumably the persistence of the leader convinces the people in the organisation that the leader can be counted on to be consistent and to act in accordance with his or her statements of strategic purpose. Also, and again presumably, the judgement that a leader can be trusted is important in the decision of people to follow her or him.

During the 1980s Kouzes and Posner (1990) investigated the types of judgements managers make about leaders in the United States. They asked over 7,500 managers from public and private sector organisations what they looked for or admired in their leaders. Four qualities stood out: the managers admired leaders who were honest, competent, forward-looking, and inspiring.

Table 2.2 Principal characteristics that US managers admire in leaders.

Characteristics of superior leaders	% of managers selecting	Meanings
Honest	87	Leaders judged by their deeds: leaders do what they say they are going to do; their behaviour is consistent with stated values and beliefs.
Competent	74	Winning track record; expertise in leadership skills; and, at higher levels, abilities in strategic planning.
Forward-looking	67	Ability to set or select a desirable destination for the organisation; convey the vision.
Inspiring	61	Enthusiastic, energetic and positive about the future.

Source: Kouzes and Posner (1990)

Kouzes and Posner noticed what they saw as a parallel between their survey results and findings about believability from research on communication. They suggested that three of the qualities they had found to be important – honesty, competence, and being inspiring – constituted being a believable or, as they called it, credible leader.

'Above all else, we must be able to believe in our leaders. We must believe that they will do what they say and that they will have the knowledge and skill to lead. They must be enthusiastic about the direction in which we are headed.'
(Kouzes and Posner 1990: 32)

Table 2.3 Believability and credibility.

Believability of sources of communication	Credibility of leaders
Trustworthy	Honest
Expertise	Competent
Dynamic	Inspiring

Source: Kouzes and Posner (1990)

Survey-based evidence suggests that managerial attitudes to leadership may be similar in the public services of the United Kingdom. The Chartered Management Institute carried out a survey of 1,890 managers in the public sector (Charlesworth *et al.* 2003). The top five attributes that public sector leaders should possess according to these managers were: clarity of vision (66 per cent), integrity (52 per cent), sound judgement (50 per cent), commitment to people development (49 per cent), and [being] strategic (46 per cent). The survey also suggested that managers thought public sector leaders should have the following skills: communicating (63 per cent), engaging employees with the vision (62 per cent), creating an enabling culture (60 per cent), formulating and implementing strategy (48 per cent), and working effectively in partnership with the community (48 per cent).

There are several obvious overlaps between these findings and those of Kouzes and Posner (1990). For example, 'integrity' and 'honesty' may be seen as related ideas. 'Sound judgement' might be associated with the idea of being 'competent'. 'Engaging employees with the vision' might be seen as the result of (and therefore linked to) being 'inspiring'.

While we have, therefore, evidence from both the United States and the United Kingdom showing that managers look to their leaders to be credible, this evidence by itself does not show that leadership credibility has effects. In essence we want to know whether the implementation of the leader's vision depends in part on 'leadership credibility'. We would expect that if leaders are credible they are believable and followers may mobilise to implement the vision. If leaders lack credibility, they are not believable and followers do not get behind the vision. The only serious and systematic investigation of the consequences of leadership credibility in the public services that we have found is a study of leadership in US local government by Gabris *et al.* (2000).

We can regard their study as building on the previous work about visionary leadership by Bennis and Nanus, and others. But the most immediate influence on their study was the research by Kouzes and Posner. They were interested in some of the usual features of visionary leadership, such as the way leaders develop a shared vision and communicate it and the way in which leaders devolve power and authority (which might be linked to empowerment). But they were also interested in whether leaders were seen as having integrity in the sense of practising what they preached, following through on promises, and generally were trusted. In their study, all of this – the visionary and the trustworthy elements of leadership – were combined together in their operationalisation of the concept of credibility. They collected data from, and on, the work of the chief administrative officer (CAO) in 11 local governments in the Chicago metropolitan area. They distributed 176 surveys to the CAOs, elected policy members, and departmental heads. The other groups were surveyed in part as a triangulation check on the data obtained from the CAOs. The CAOs were mayors, city managers, or city administrators.

The researchers used the surveys to investigate the 'leadership credibility' of the CAOs and they used eight items in the surveys to measure it.

1 The CAO clearly communicates the purpose and rationale behind new programmes and reforms.
2 The CAO actively works to communicate the organisation's vision and mission to employees.
3 The development of a shared vision and set of core values is a fundamental objective of the CAO.
4 Employees believe they can trust the CAO and put their fate in his/her hands.
5 The CAO makes sure employees have sufficient power and authority to accomplish assigned objectives.
6 The CAO practises what he/she preaches in terms of values, work effort, and reform. The CAO sets a good example.
7 The CAO follows through on promises regarding changes others are expected to carry out.
8 The CAO actively seeks to reward, praise, and recognise high performance.

Clearly they were using the concept of credibility to mean much more than the existence of trust in leadership. As we have noted, it also represents the idea of visionary leadership in the sense that it refers to the development of shared vision and the communication of vision by the leader. It also addresses the issue of employees having sufficient power and authority to make decisions, which might be seen as indicative of an effective practice of empowerment. It also contains a transactional element – the leader recognising and rewarding high performance.

They compared the data from elected officials, the CAOs and the departmental managers and they used Cronbach's alpha coefficients to check on the reliability of their measure of leadership credibility. These checks reassured them that they had a reliable measure. But, did leadership credibility matter? Gabris and his co-researchers reported statistical correlations between their measure of the leadership credibility of the CAO and the performance of the local government organisation. Both how well the organisation adapted to its environment and the overall effectiveness of the organisation as a service and program provider were correlated with the CAO leadership credibility measure.

Table 2.4 Leadership credibility and local government performance.

Variable	Simple product-moment correlation with leadership credibility
This organisation adapts well to its environment	0.59
The overall effectiveness of this local government organisation as a service and program provider	0.60

Note: Both correlations were significant at the 0.1 level using a one-tailed test.
Source: Gabris et al. (2000: 100 and 105)

Alban-Metcalfe and Alimo-Metcalfe (2000) have also contributed some interesting evidence on the importance of honesty and integrity and have reported some effects of such leadership attributes in their UK study of nearly 1,500 local government managers. They used principal components analysis to identify nine factors that they described as forming the basis of scales reflecting transformational aspects of leadership. They labelled one of these scales as 'Integrity, trustworthy, honest and open'. The specific items in this scale are: 'makes it easy for me to admit mistakes', 'is trustworthy', and 'takes decisions based on moral and ethical principles'. This scale was found to correlate with three dependent variables: job satisfaction, satisfying leadership style, and (inversely) stress. We would underline the obvious overlap here with the honesty element in the Kouzes and Posner concept of credibility.

To sum up, we have an interesting leadership concept in the idea of credibility. This is so, in our opinion, whether we see it as a composite of a set of qualities (honest, competent, and inspiring) or as a fusion of visionary leadership, trustworthiness, devolution of power and authority, and transactional attention to recognising and rewarding those who are high performers. We would add that the concept of leadership credibility is, in our opinion, useful because it serves to raise doubts about the easy identity between the action of a leader producing a vision and action by empowered employees. Under certain conditions the vision may lead easily into successful empowered action by followers. But, if there is a problem about the believability of the leaders, will followers act in an empowered way? Based on Gabris *et al.*'s work (2000), the answer is probably not. We can take this speculation a little further: if the followers do feel empowered to act to implement the vision, but the leaders have unsound judgement causing the vision to be wrong, it might also be assumed that there will be subsequent damage to the credibility of the leaders.

Effects on followers

The notion that leaders affect people by empowering them is an attractive idea. We would have liked to look directly at detailed evidence from studies of empowerment, which is defined by us as occurring when people are invited to share responsibility for making the organisation's vision come true and when they accept this responsibility and act accordingly using their initiative. But the published research on the public services has so far provided little detailed understanding of the nature of empowerment and what encourages and shapes it.

Above we suggested that leadership credibility intervenes between the vision of the leader and empowerment, and thus modifies the effects that leaders have. What else modifies the effects of leaders on followers? And what else can leaders do to reinforce the importance of the vision and its implementation? We cannot fully answer these questions, but we will consider some evidence that is suggestive of important conditions in terms of the impact leaders have on those they lead.

It is possible that in the UK, perhaps in contrast to North America, leadership effects depend on the followers seeing a degree of reciprocity in the relationship with leaders. This suggestion is prompted by the work of Alban-Metcalfe and Alimo-Metcalfe (2000). They reported that their study of nearly 1,500 UK local government managers had found that a leadership factor that they labelled as 'Genuine Concern for Others' was the best predictor of five criterion variables. The data, gathered by a questionnaire, asked managers about a manager or colleague with whom they had worked closely. They were interested in the phenomenon of 'nearby' or 'close' transformational leadership at different levels. The leadership factor they identified included items referring to 'genuine interest in me as an individual' and 'develops my strengths'. The criterion variables were: enabling more achievement than expected, motivation to achieve more than expected, satisfaction with leadership style, job satisfaction, and job-related stress. The last variable, job-related stress, was, as might be guessed, inversely related to 'Genuine Concern for Others'. We are obviously suggesting that followers respond positively to a belief that nearby leaders care about them. If nearby leaders are not perceived as being concerned about others perhaps this inhibits a sense of responsibility developing among followers, which shows up as depressed motivation to achieve and less actual achievement than expected.

Some of their later work with data for over 4,000 managers in the UK also suggested that the leadership model of UK public services also corresponded reasonably well with a model for the UK private sector. They found that a leader's concern for individuals' well-being and development was pre-eminent in both sectors. To quote them, they found 'a virtually identical model of leadership in both the public and private sectors in the UK' (Alimo-Metcalfe and Alban Metcalfe 2002: 34).

Perhaps empowerment is sustained by the hope of being rewarded. The empirical research on credibility by Gabris and his colleagues included in the concept of credibility the idea that leaders recognise and reward people who perform well. They were influenced by Kouzes and Posner, who believed that leadership credibility can be built up, and who suggested that there were ten learnable commitments, one of which was described as 'recognise individual contribution'.

We think there is yet another study where it might be inferred that extra effort (and thus perhaps increased empowerment) is created or sustained by rewards. This is a study by Gellis (2001) of transformational leadership among hospital social workers. A questionnaire was given out to 234 social workers in 26 hospitals and some 187 were returned completed (i.e. 80 per cent response rate). The questionnaire had been based on the Multifactor Leadership Questionnaire (Bass and Avolio 1990) and the social workers were asked about their direct managers. This study was carried out at a time when the hospitals were being affected by major reforms in the health sector and this was causing major changes in service delivery. Statistical analysis (using Pearson Product-Moment correlations) showed that the five transformational subscales but only one of the transactional subscales were related to three outcome variables, including a measure of extra effort by the social worker. This is shown in Figure 2.1.

Gellis gives as an example of 'idealized influence attributed' an item that refers to going beyond self-interest for the good of a group. 'Idealized influence behaviours' is illustrated using an item relating to the importance of having a strong sense of purpose. Inspirational motivation is concerned with the communication of a vision. Individualised consideration involves the leader in paying attention to employee needs and helping employees learn through responsibility. Intellectual stimulation is about providing new ideas that can be used by employees to find new ways of doing things.

Gellis then applied a hierarchical regression procedure by first entering the transactional leadership behaviours and then adding in the transformational leadership behaviour factors. This increased the explained variance for the outcome variables. Gellis concluded that transformational leadership was associated with higher levels of extra effort and satisfaction as compared to transactional leadership by itself.

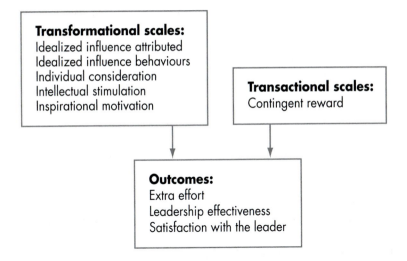

Figure 2.1 Gellis's study of transformational leadership among hospital social workers.

But the point remains that contingent rewards are a factor in explaining leadership effectiveness, effort made, and leader satisfaction. Perhaps, therefore, contingent reward is an important factor in empowerment?

We think it is worth noting that these findings showed that the best result is obtained when managers use both transactional and transformational leadership. This is reminiscent of Gabris *et al.*'s formulation of credible leadership such that it includes a leader actively seeking to reward, praise and recognise performance (see above) as well as communicating a vision. It would seem, therefore, that transactional behaviour (contingent rewards) and transformational leadership behaviour should both co-exist to get the best results.

Finally, do leaders simply hope that their persuasive abilities are sufficient to ensure that action by those they lead will be oriented to the realisation of the vision, or do they have ways of affecting employees to reinforce the direction they want the organisation to go in? In other words do leaders have any other ways of ensuring positive outcomes apart from their communication of the vision?

Bennis and Nanus (1985) argue that the vision has to be embedded and sustained. Leaders work at reinforcing the vision through strategic decision-making and through culture management. The latter is very important – change often requires leaders to help managers and employees to undergo the cultural change required if the organisation is to adapt to new circumstances (Heifetz and Linsky 2002).

Kouzes and Posner's (1990) work provides some suggestive evidence consistent with the importance of strategic decision-making to leadership. Three-quarters of the 7,500 managers from public and private sector organisations that they surveyed selected as a crucial characteristic of leaders that they should be 'competent' and two-thirds of managers selected the characteristic of being 'forward-looking'. They suggested that leaders at higher levels are expected to demonstrate competence through strategic planning abilities. They also (1990: 31) commented: 'Forward-looking does not mean possessing the magical power of a visionary. The reality is far more down-to-earth. It is the ability to set or select a desirable destination for the organization.' So it might be argued that being able to do strategic planning and set strategic direction are important attributes sought by people in their leaders.

In another report on their work Alimo-Metcalfe and Alban-Metcalfe (2002) present a model of leadership for the public sector that has 12 leadership scales based on data from more than 3,500 participating individual managers. In this case, one of the scales refers to the leader as having 'a clear vision and strategic direction'. This could be seen as implying that leaders need to be good at strategic thinking.

We have already referred above to the study by Gabris *et al.* (2000) of credible leaders in local government. They also reported evidence of a statistical association between leadership credibility (LC) of the chief administration officer and the use by a local government of more advanced strategic planning techniques. They concluded (Gabris *et al.* 2000: 99): 'Overall, then, LC seems to be reasonably associated with enhanced perceptions about the local government's strategic capacity, as expected.' They also found a statistical association between leadership credibility and support for the statement that strategic changes were constantly a priority.

This last study provides evidence of a possible link between strategic planning and leadership. The findings, if not conclusive, are at least consistent with the idea that leaders use strategic decision-making to reinforce their effectiveness as leaders. Moreover, if leadership works in large part by motivating managers and employees to pursue the implementation of a vision and creating a state of empowerment, then strategic decision-making and culture management may be seen as ways of focusing empowerment.

To sum up, on the basis of the evidence currently available, leadership charisma may seem very glamorous but its 'cash value' would appear to be a lot less certain than the more prosaic concept of leadership credibility. So instead of hankering after a mysterious personal quality, public services leaders should concentrate on building their credibility. This may be seen as centred on personal integrity, sound judgement, and being inspirational, or, on the basis of the work by Gabris *et al.*, it may be seen as centred on visionary leadership, trust, devolved power, and recognition and rewards for high levels of performance. Empowerment of managers and employees is probably not purely based on activating some higher common purpose. We have suggested that a perception of reciprocity in the relationship with leaders and recognition and rewards by leaders are probably important. There is probably a transactional element in even the notion of being inspired to transform an organisation. The leader does not merely communicate the vision and then stand back – the vision has to be embedded, sustained, and focused. This may be done through strategic decision-making and through culture management (and cultural change).

OTHER MANAGEMENT LEADERS

The idea that leaders develop more leaders has been around for quite some time. Follett suggested that the best leader worked not merely to create multiple leaders in his or her organisation but also to combine them effectively:

> 'If the best leader takes all the means in his power to develop leadership among his subordinates and gives them opportunity to exercise it, he has then his supreme task, to unite all the different degrees and different types of leadership that come to the surface in the ramifications of a modern business.'
>
> (Follett 1941: 282)

Where there are multiple leaders in an organisation, therefore, there is an issue about how leaders create and relate to a network of leaders. There is no reason to suppose that all leaders relate in the same way to any such network of leaders in their organisation. But there is anecdotal evidence that leaders at the top of an organisation can value a leadership network for bringing about radical change. Osborne and Gaebler (1992) attributed a turnaround of Tactical Air Command of the US Air Force to a General Creech, and they quoted him as saying that there had been a decentralisation of responsibility as well as authority and 'a new spirit of leadership' appeared 'at many levels'.

Pettigrew *et al.*'s (1992) study of strategic change in the UK's National Health Service analysed leadership in terms of groups, teams, collectivities, and cabals. In respect of one case study they wrote: 'The key group which in the end achieved change was not part of the mainstream planning machinery but a rather odd and informal "study group" with no chairman and no clinical representative . . . the construction and maintenance of such teams must be an important issue' (Pettigrew *et al.* 1992: 99). The dispersed nature of leadership was also identified in two further cases studied by Pettigrew and his co-researchers (Pettigrew *et al.* 1992: 215): 'The common denominator in Huddersfield and Mid Downs was the way the leadership of change was shared across a caucus of people.' There were differences between the cases. In Huddersfield the researchers found a critical mass of enthusiasts who formed a powerful team for the delivery of change, but in the Mid Downs case the 'power house for change' was a smaller and tighter group of key people. It is also noteworthy that in the Huddersfield case, which had been characterised by the use of ad-hoc groups and informal communications, there were some people who felt excluded from an inner 'cabal'. Possibly this shows that when an informal coalition of enthusiasts brings about change, the informality and improvised nature of group decision-making is more prone to criticism of exclusiveness in decision-making.

We conclude that leadership of change in big public services organisations is often not confined to a single person at the top level – leadership may be provided by a team of people or a coalition of leaders at one or more organisational levels.

MANAGERIAL LEADERS AND ELECTED POLITICIANS AND CITIZENS

As reported above, Alban-Metcalfe and Alimo-Metcalfe (2000) analysed data from nearly 1,500 local government managers and used principal components analysis to identify nine factors, including one they labelled 'political sensitivity and skills'. This consisted of items about being sensitive to the political pressures on elected politicians, understanding dynamics of the leading group amongst the elected politicians, and being able to work with elected politicians to achieve results. This particular scale appeared not to be that interesting in terms of explaining the achievements and motivation to achieve of the managers, but it is possible that managerial leaders possessing such political skills might be important for other reasons.

Gabris *et al.* (2000) reported finding a strong correlation between the leadership credibility of the chief administrative officers and reports of their being effective in their interactions with elected policy board members in US local government. Likewise they reported there was a strong correlation between leadership credibility and the perception that the chief administrative officer was effective in his external actions, for example, with citizens. These findings suggest that political skills in relation to elected politicians and external stakeholders could well be an important aspect of public services leadership credibility. We are tempted to suggest that public services leaders who are perceived to have such political skills are more likely to be believable as leaders. This seems logical. The leader who has political skills should enjoy more political support and thus achieve more success in implementing strategic plans (Heymann 1987).

MANAGERIAL LEADERS AND PARTNERS

As we have already noted above, Alban-Metcalfe and Alimo-Metcalfe's (2000) analysis of data from a sample of nearly 1,500 UK local government managers led to the identification of a number of leadership scales. One of these was 'inspirational networker and promoter'. They explained the meaning of this scale through linking it to the following items:

- has a wide network of links to external environment;
- effectively promotes the work/achievements of the department/ organisation to the outside world;
- is able to communicate the vision of the authority/department to the public/community.

All three of these items can plausibly be seen as important in partnership working with the community. However, the researchers performed a stepwise multiple-regression and this showed that this leadership scale in the UK sample was mostly not important in predicting outcome variables. Only in the case of employees reporting that the leader had a satisfying leadership style was there any evidence that being an inspirational networker and promoter mattered.

Alimo-Metcalfe and Alban-Metcalfe's (2002) work on a dataset of over 4,000 managers, most of who worked in the public sector, presented a more complex picture of public sector leadership. Again as we have already noted, they reported 14 leadership scales for the public sector leaders and two of them made reference to external stakeholders:

- Inspiring communicator of the vision of the organisation to a network of internal and external stakeholders; gains the confidence and support of various groups through sensitivity to needs and by achieving organisational goals.
- Has a clear vision and strategic direction; engages various internal and external stakeholders in developing; helps others to achieve the vision.

There is case study evidence on partnership working with the community from the Frost-Kumpf *et al.* (1993) study of successful transformational change at Ohio Department of Mental Health (ODMH). In this case, the importance of the partnership process appears to have been to gain access to ideas (Frost-Kumpf *et al.* 1993: 142–3): 'By deliberately sharing power with consumers and other constituency groups, the leaders of ODMH gained access to new information and ideas.' This point is repeated (1993: 144): 'Between 1983 and 1986, the leadership of ODMH worked strenuously to develop, involve, and empower key constituency groups. For example, numerous regional, statewide, and national conferences were held, involving members of various constituency groups throughout Ohio.'

EVALUATION

It is unlikely that the preceding research findings will come as much of a surprise to anyone who has read any of the literature in the last two decades about visionary leadership and transformational leadership.

(1) The findings do seem to confirm Kotter's (2001) view of leadership action as concerned with vision and strategies, communicating, motivating and inspiring and getting people to align themselves with vision and values. If we take managers to be concerned with producing order, organising people, designing organisations, planning and solving problems (Kotter 2001), then we can note that this set of research findings suggests little overlap of the role of leader with the role of manager.

It is tempting to suggest that a visionary leadership model for the public services can be presented in a diagrammatic form showing a process of empowerment to produce innovation and transformation, which is then maintained through a set of reinforcing actions by leaders or stimulated by leadership behaviour.

(2) But one surprising finding is the lack of clear-cut differences in leadership between the private and public sectors. Bennis and Nanus

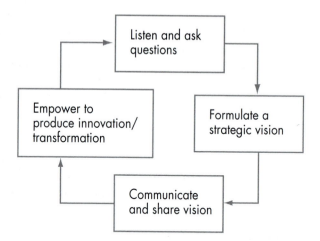

Reinforcing actions by leaders:
Act as role models for personal learning
Raise energy levels
Distribute leadership to groups, coalitions, and networks of leaders
Develop the organisation and show genuine concern for people in the organisation
Recognise and reward good performance
Embed and sustain vision through strategic decision-making and culture management

Figure 2.2 A model of visionary leadership in the public services.

(1985) had data on leaders from both sectors but did not report differences according to sector. In the case of UK research by Alimo-Metcalfe and Alban-Metcalfe, there is an explicit claim that the models of leadership for the two sectors are virtually identical. But it is still possible that research has inadvertently concentrated on similarities between leadership in the two sectors and there remain to be discovered important differences related to sector.

(3) We now move on to some potential problems with the theory of visionary leadership. The first of these is that it presents the process of leadership in a very idealistic way. Each step in the process is identified – from listening and asking questions through to empowerment – but do transitions from one part of the leadership process to another always proceed smoothly and unhindered? Or are there blockages and disruptions that occur sufficiently frequently that they deserve attention in any theory of leadership? We think the answer must be that there are. The research on leadership credibility helps to create a more realistic model of visionary leadership in which the translation of vision through empowerment into action is much more problematic.

(4) The studies by Alimo-Metcalfe and Alban-Metcalfe in the UK (2001, 2003) have in some respects suggested either that the model of visionary leadership is only applicable to some leaders or that it is much more complex than might be so far supposed. They warn us to look again carefully at the idea that the most important thing about leaders is that they articulate and share a strategic vision. In the case of a sample of nearly 1,500 local government managers, Alimo-Metcalfe and Alban-Metcalfe (2003) found 14 different dimensions of leadership, including one they labelled as 'building a shared vision'. They also suggested that in the case of male managers there was a link between this dimension and the respondent's reported motivation to achieve. However, this link was not found for middle managers or female managers.

(5) The same researchers, commenting on their analysis of UK data on over 4,000 public sector and private sector managers, have raised the possibility that there are UK and US differences in leadership (Alimo-Metcalfe and Alban-Metcalfe 2002: 34):

'The British model was more complex and revealed that the most important issue for managers in both [private and public] sectors was concern for individuals' well-being and development. US models identify the two top leadership characteristics as vision and charisma – qualities that are ranked much lower by UK managers . . . while the emphasis in the US is on the leader as role model, our study suggests that the most important pre-requisite for a leader is what they can do for their staff. This is far more similar to the model of the leader as a servant.'

This speculation is interesting but it is just speculation. It is possible that differences between their British studies and US findings might be explained by their research design and the sample they used. For example, they were asking about 'near leaders' and they were asking people we might term 'followers'. Perhaps the immediate followers of any leader are more likely than anyone else to stress that they want a leader who is sensitive to their needs and interests.

But what if we take the differences suggested by Alimo-Metcalfe and Alban-Metcalfe at face value? What if effective US leaders are more visionary and UK leaders are more likely to be effective if they show genuine concern for individuals' well-being and development? Perhaps it shows that UK public services employees are more transactional or less trusting of their leaders? Perhaps they need more convincing of the existence of reciprocity in the relationship between leaders and led?

A NORMATIVE MODEL OF LEADERSHIP

A recent survey reported by Charlesworth *et al.* (2003) shows us the opinions of a large number of UK public sector managers and we would expect that their opinions would to some appreciable degree reflect reality. Consequently we can draw up a normative model of public services leadership, a model showing what public services managers think their leaders should do.

While this model has been shaped out of the findings on what public sector managers say leaders should do or be good at, it is also influenced by Philip Heymann's (1987) studies of strategic management in the United States. Hence the theming of the findings reflects Heymann's argument that successful strategy in the public sector is based on a vision of the needs to be met, the development of the necessary organisational capacity, and the development of the necessary

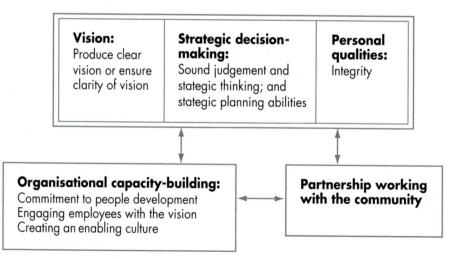

Figure 2.3 A normative model of leadership based on a UK survey of public sector managers.

external support. This model brings out the importance of partnership working with the community that is not emphasised in the usual accounts of visionary leadership.

CONCLUSIONS

What lessons for public services leaders can be distilled from the research we have reviewed?

First, there is evidence that leadership in public services organisations is important in finding and clarifying a strategic vision to act as a target for strategic change. The evidence currently points to the importance of the leader in ensuring the vision exists and is clear. It does not place on the leader the responsibility for dreaming it up or originating a vision.

Secondly, leaders communicate and share the vision and this then can lead to action by others who see new possibilities of action as a result of the speeches and statements of leaders.

Thirdly, in terms of personal qualities, there is evidence that leaders need to be honest, have integrity and be inspiring, as well as be capable of using sound judgement. Words such as 'trustworthy' and 'credible' were prominent in the work on the personal qualities of public services leaders. There is little reason on the basis of the research published to date to suggest that public services leaders need to have charisma if they are to be successful.

Fourthly, leaders who express their 'genuine interest in staff as individuals' and/or demonstrate 'individualised consideration' have more effect on their followers.

Fifthly, leaders in the public services need political skills in order to be credible leaders.

Sixthly, the best results are obtained when inspirational leaders who develop and share strategic visions are also making sure that they recognise and reward good performance.

Seventhly, another point to have emerged from the research findings is the view that models of leadership are not substantially different between the public and private sectors. This is the clear conclusion from the studies by Beverley Alimo-Metcalfe and John Alban-Metcalfe. Although there were some minor differences between leadership in the two sectors, the more striking conclusion is their similarity.

Finally, Beverley Alimo-Metcalfe and John Alban-Metcalfe have pointed to differences between UK and US studies. Variations in sampling or methods used (data collection and analysis) might have caused differences. However, if this is a real difference, it might be that UK leaders place less emphasis on vision and charisma and more on doing things for their employees' well-being and development. If this is so, it might suggest that the type of leadership that is dominant reflects contextual factors. So, in the case of Britain leaders may need to demonstrate a greater concern for reciprocity in their relations with followers. If we combine it with the preceding observation about the apparent lack of a sectoral difference in leadership, it suggests that national culture or circumstances matter more than differences in the private sector and public sector environments.

CHAPTER 3

IN SEARCH OF LEADERSHIP

MYTHS AND CONUNDRUMS

Perusal of airport bookshops can leave one in little doubt that a manifest obsession amongst those who have an interest in organisations and their management, is that of leadership. The titles one might find range from the inspirational to the mechanistic but all reflect thematic priorities developed in research-based literature and echoed by politicians across the globe – that the search for leadership is deemed to be a key determinant of organisational success regardless of sector.

Yet there is a degree of paradox associated with this apparently ever-increasing spotlight being turned upon the importance of leadership and indeed of leaders *per se* being the key attribute in attaining and sustaining organisational transformation and success. For if we consider that management theories are at least in part evolutionary, then this emphasis upon the apparent key role of individuals at the very top of organisations, sits somewhat uncomfortably with the emphasis placed upon teams and group capacity for learning and innovation that was dominant in the 1980s and 1990s. Has there been a major step-change in organisational thinking and prioritisation? Or are we now seeing a cyclical process whereby leadership, which has arguably been a key point of discussion and debate since the history of mankind was first chronicled, is once more moving centre stage? It is possible of course to posit a view that the answer to these two questions lies at some mid-point – that quality management, performance management and organisational learning have all been hugely influential is undoubtedly true; however, their capacity for delivering sustained and organic change and a real sense of organisational renewal, is perhaps less categorically proven. Therefore, a sense of 'gap' has developed and into this the predominance of leadership as a key organisational aspiration has taken hold.

Senge, reflecting upon the rise of leadership and its paradoxical juxtapositioning around aspirations to have less hierarchical organisational structures, points to lack of maturity and confidence in organisations as being a key driver in the push for visible leadership:

'... the myth of the omnipotent CEO is merely a special case of a deeper cultural icon, the myth of the hero-leader. According to this shared story, leaders are the few special people blessed with the capability for command and influence. They have become leaders precisely because of their unique mix of skill, ambition, vision, charisma, and no small amount of hubris. They can overcome the blocks that stymie everyone else. They make great things happen. The implication is clear: if you too want to make a difference, you had better be one of these special people.'

(Senge 1999: 10)

So what are we to make of this person specification? Senge, although largely reflecting upon commercial sector settings, identifies themes and priorities that characterise senior-level public service appointment advertisements across many countries. Clearly such people are likely to be rare indeed, and for those who have built up careers over time in a public service environment, the requirement to exemplify highly visible capacity for 'command and influence', may be at some variance from the traditions and behaviours with which they developed. Fenlon suggests that those holding senior public service roles have some uniquely challenging issues to contend with:

'While private sector executives are concerned with growing profits that exceed the cost of capital, public sector executives must focus on producing benefits that exceed the cost of political capital, which is the breadth and depth of support possessed by a leader. Besides this they must utilise financial and social measures of performance.

Public sector executives face a variety of obstacles and challenges when implementing strategies. For example, measures of success and service effectiveness are notoriously difficult to establish making evaluation and accountability problematic. In addition, public sector executives face unique obstacles in leading organisational change, in part because of entrenched civil service bureaucracies, procedural constraints such as managing performance and firing employees, and dealing with many different stakeholders with competing priorities.'

(Fenlon 2002: 4)

Thus, Fenlon has set out some of the key differences and challenges facing those holding or indeed aspiring to hold senior-level positions within the public service environment. To fundamentally understand them and their complexity is central to any real understanding of the functions and limitations of leadership and leadership theories that may be applied within this diverse and evolving 'sector'. These critical areas of focus provide much of the structure and many of the thematic priorities for this chapter:

- Leadership is seen across a range of sectoral settings. Fenlon's articulation of a view that there is considerable divergence between commercial and public service settings appears defensible but does require some further testing, particularly in respect of the concepts of *management* and *leadership* and the degree of overlap that there may be around the two areas.

- The apparent absence of an overt profit motive as being something that once again serves to potentially differentiate the style of leadership required. This too is an assertion which requires careful testing, particularly in respect of emergent models of 'public service' offering which are subject to market testing and competition from third party providers. Certainly this *market* scenario, whilst largely immature, is one which is increasingly influential and potentially adds yet a further requirement to the specification outlined by Senge; to everything else might now potentially be added the need to display entrepreneurial tendencies.

- Performance measurement and an agenda of accountability represent key areas that any investigation of public service leadership must demonstrate proper awareness of. Where measures are potentially so qualitatively and also politically driven, to what extent is there the capacity for the type of creative leadership that Senge refers to, actually to develop and flourish?

- Critically the above point steers our focus towards the critical role of politics and of politicians within the public service leadership domain. Public service leaders have no more important stakeholders than those who hold and influence political power, it is from them that they derive policy priorities, strategic imperatives and targets to be held accountable against. The extent to which political agendas and time-frames impact upon the ability of public service organisations to be led differentially – i.e. in ways which are innovative and creative – represents a critical area of concern.

- The concept of leader-delivered change almost presupposes an organisational capacity and willingness to do so. Yet public service operating structures even today, after a period of some decades of often profound reform, retain bureaucratic and cultural traits that make them difficult environments in which to seek to drive forward a meaningful change agenda. A question that on occasions needs to be asked is, are public service organisations receptive to the concept of being led?

In moving forward to consider the detailed areas outlined above it is important to draw this section to a conclusion by returning to the concept of leadership as having the potential to have many myths associated with it and so many allied layers of complexity as to make it one of the most challenging areas of study in modern organisational thinking. In discussing the mythology of leadership, Senge argues that in organisations today:

'The word "leader" has become a synonym for top manager. When people talk about "developing leaders" they mean developing prospective top managers. When they ask, "What do the leaders think?" they ask the views of the top managers.

There are two problems with this. First, it implies that those who are not in top management positions are not leaders. They might aspire to "become" leaders, but they don't get there until they reach a senior management position of authority. Second, it leaves us with no real definition of leadership. If leadership is simply a position in the hierarchy, then, in effect, there is no independent definition of leadership.'

(Senge 1999: 16)

Thus, for Senge at least, the neo-classical view of leadership as being associated with seniority is a perspective that is ripe for challenge. Yet to do so, it may be argued, requires an organisational culture and a wider operating environment that truly does seek to devolve authority and responsibility away from a central focus. As we shall discuss later in this chapter, there may be many tensions that militate against such an approach being always entirely possible within many of the extant public service environments that may be observed.

Goffee and Jones, whilst broadly allying themselves with the position that Senge argues for so forcefully, do provide further insight into the scope of key tensions that can be observed in organisations today; these they categorise as the four most common leadership myths:

'**1. Everyone can be a leader**. Not true. Many executives don't have the self-knowledge or the authenticity for leadership. At the same time, self-knowledge and authenticity are necessary but not sufficient conditions for leadership. Individuals must also want to be leaders, and many perfectly talented employees are not interested in shouldering that responsibility.

2. Leaders deliver successful business results. Not always. Some well-led businesses do not necessarily produce short-term results, while some businesses with successful results are not necessarily well led. If results were always a matter of good leadership, picking leaders would be easy.

3. People who get to the top are leaders. Not necessarily. One of the most persistent misperceptions is that people in leadership positions are leaders. But people who make it to the top may have done so because of political acumen, not necessarily true leadership quality. What's more, real leaders are found all over the organisation, from the executive suite to the shop floor. By definition, leaders are simply people who have followers – and rank doesn't have much to do with that. Effective military organisations have long realised the importance of developing leaders at many levels.

4. Leaders are great coaches. Rarely. A whole cottage industry has grown up around the idea that good leaders ought to be good coaches. But this belief rests on the assumption that a single person can both inspire the troops and impart technical skills.'

(Goffee and Jones 2002: 4)

Leadership, it would appear, is characterised by largely mercurial characteristics. It can be everywhere in an organisation, it can be largely absent, and yet neither extreme provides an absolute indicator of likely success. Crainer, in reviewing definitions of leadership, put aside his scholarly search having found some 400 which he felt were defensible and his caution that theoretical perspectives represent 'a veritable minefield of misunderstanding through which . . . practitioners must tread warily', is a wise one (Crainer 1996: xiii).

In seeking to consider how the complexities of leadership as a concept translate into the public service environment it is worthwhile reflecting upon the perspective set out by Sir Peter Parker, as a leader and manager perhaps best known for his seven-year tenure as Chairman of British Rail – the United Kingdom's pre-privatisation national rail network. In Parker's view successful leadership in public service organisations should be characterised by a clear focus on three key dimensions – the *economic,* the *entrepreneurial* and the *social* (Parker 1989: 3). By the economic we can take him to mean the requirement to achieve focus upon all aspects of performance, from the general acceptance of a requirement to deliver balanced and surplus generating operating budgets, through to the focus upon key aspects of service provision allied to targets and service level agreements. His emphasis upon the entrepreneurial traits of leadership is firmly focused upon the development of organisational capacity to innovate and change, for leaders to be fundamentally focused upon challenging any sense of *status quo.* For Parker, the social dimension to public service leadership was held to be absolutely key in terms of attracting, motivating and retaining the best people. Having a capacity to focus upon leading for a 'public good', to seek improvements based upon something other than a bottom-line profit agenda, is potentially the single greatest area of difference that sets apart the plethora of generalist definitions of leadership from a more public service specific model. As Fenlon argues:

'I have drawn the rather paradoxical conclusion that public and private leadership is fundamentally alike and different in important respects. The essentials of leadership and management in the public sector are the same as those in the private sector. Yet, public sector executives also confront unique challenges in every aspect of their leadership.'

(Fenlon 2002: 4)

BUT WE ARE DIFFERENT . . .

The possibility that leadership styles and traits must be essentially different with the public services is a contentious view – certainly many politicians from Margaret Thatcher onwards have lamented that public service behaviours and cultures do not exhibit greater synergy with those found in commercial sector settings. It is possible to argue, and many have done so of course, that this is a highly subjective and politicised view which seeks to establish polarities – to posit a black and white, good and bad, if you will, view of the world of management and leadership.

It is important also to seek out anecdotes which may serve to provide additional perspective upon such views. One such 'story' emanates from a world-renowned business school offering both generalist MBA programmes and more specialist programmes in public administration. Analysis of their applications and admissions over the period 1997–2002 suggested that public service organisation sponsorship of employees to attend such programmes had grown exponentially and that, interestingly, most of these new students were opting for generalist over specialist programmes. What does this tell us? Fundamentally there is the possibility for both positive and cynical interpretation of such an informal report – the first perspective might suggest that a key lesson learned for public service personnel is that they are rather less different in their practices and development needs than they might have anticipated and acknowledge this through their programme choices. A rather more cynical interpretation is that such sponsored personnel are rather keener to enhance their own personal marketability and may have no underpinning commitment to a public service career.

Anecdotes aside, what is clear in any analysis of the public service environment is that by its very nature and mission, it will be different from that which might be observed in the commercial sector. However, the intention here is to challenge the sense of *absolutism*, which might view the two areas as having no meaningful correlation in their requirements and practices. It is possible to argue that there are a number of unquestionable points of overlap, where the differences will be those of context rather than profound sectoral disconnection. The first of these meeting-points must surely be an agreed position that sees all sectors within an economy recognising the need for the complementary traits of management and leadership to be deployed successfully. Within this paradigm of complementarity, we see the role of leadership as being essential in developing and communicating organisational mission and strategies; motivating all key stakeholders to take on ownership of the organisational future; and, critically, to be viewed as the key locus for change and renewal within the organisation. The management function therefore exists to ensure that the structures, processes, people and systems required to deliver organisational success are in place and are regularly monitored.

Consideration of the leadership-management model offers us both a defensible and a logical frame of reference for our consideration of the extent to which the public service might diverge from any agreed position. To further contextualise this position it is useful to reflect upon the case of the New York City Police Department (NYPD). Now one of the most often used examples in leadership development programmes across all sectors, the NYPD example serves to provide some significant insights into the key differences which we might posit in respect of a public service leadership agenda:

'The New York City Police Department (NYPD) brought in new leaders after the election of Rudolph Giuliani as New York mayor in 1993. They set a direction for the department that produced dramatic benefits for the public, exceeding the cost of political capital employed.

From the 1960s onward, the department's leaders confronted spiralling violence and drug-related crime. In the early 1990s, the city was averaging over 2,000 murders a year. A national magazine ran a cover image of New York City, mocking the "big apple" as the "rotting apple", and portraying the decline that many New Yorkers had come to accept as impervious to reform effects. The department itself, the largest municipal agency in the US, was demoralised. A survey conducted at the time revealed that officers were more concerned about staying out of trouble than fighting crime.

In the face of this challenge and the many obstacles to changing a massive, entrenched public-service organisation, leaders developed new strategies that transformed all aspects of the organisation, including structure, culture, use of technology, measures and rewards and bringing new people into leadership roles.

Giuliani and department leaders adopted the "broken windows theory", which links minor crime and lawlessness to more serious crime. They introduced new strategies to enhance the quality of life in the city by concentrating on relatively minor violations such as graffiti, panhandling and street-level drug dealing. These aggressive policing strategies exacted certain costs of political capital. For example, some community activists protested that these strategies fostered unjustifiably intrusive or even abusive behaviour by police.

Yet as the city came under control, and as rates for serious crimes like murder and rape began to fall dramatically, particularly in the poorest neighbourhoods with the highest crime rates, the benefits outweighed the costs of political capital incurred by the department and Giuliani.

Police leaders increased accountability in the force via a new measurement system called the CompStat programme. Prior to this, the main measure of success was the number of arrests made by a unit. As leaders clarified the department's mission, which was not to make arrests but to reduce crime, the new accountability system provided a way of measuring progress against this goal.

The programme created transparency as every precinct commander began to measure a variety of crime data on a daily basis (rather than waiting for FBI crime statistics) including civilian complaints about the force itself. Sophisticated analysis let commanders pinpoint and respond to sudden shifts in crime patterns. Individual commanders had to attend forums with leaders and peers to present their data, defend practices, share learning and obtain input.

The CompStat programme helped the NYPD address two leadership challenges in the public sector: measuring results and accountability. The results were dramatic: New York City fell to 160th place on the FBI's city list for crime in the US in 2000. While the new strategies under Giuliani incurred some costs in political capital, the new direction dramatically reduced crime – what William Bratton, police commissioner, called the public-sector equivalent of profit.'

(Giuliani 2002: 62)

The transformation of an organisation as exemplified by the NYPD, from a position of being reactive and governed by outdated practices, into one which is, if nothing else, characterised by its proactive and forward-looking agenda, demonstrates perfectly the positive alignment of leadership and management forces. To a very great extent, and undoubtedly one of the reasons why this is a case that is used so frequently across sectoral divides, the issues that are raised are common to all sectors. Achievement of clear focus upon mission, together with effective and properly informed leadership, is an aspiration for organisations as diverse as those concerned with the provision of social care and those seeking to maximise profit in the sale of insurance.

However, in one important respect, the Giuliani case gives us some insight into two areas of key difference which can legitimately be argued to set apart the public service environment. The first of these is the reference to the importance of recognising costs to *political capital*, and although aspects of this will be developed later in this chapter it is worth emphasising the importance of understanding and acknowledging the existence of such a concept here. Political capital derives from the 'balance sheet' or 'workbook' approach that is extant in the minds of almost all democratically elected leaders – put simply, a positive entry on to such a 'sheet' would reflect the positive impact upon an individual and/or an administration arising from the development and implementation of a policy. And, as with all double entry accounting methods, where there is a facility for recording the positive, there must, even perhaps more critically, be some mechanism for ensuring that the negative consequences of an action are properly understood and factored into developmental thinking.

In the case of the NYPD, it was possible to observe an organisation in crisis that was then exposed to a high degree of political leadership – which articulated a view around mission and purpose and required all those involved in leading on the operational issues to mirror new imperatives through their own styles, behaviours and expectations. However, a key question to ask here in respect of seeking to differentiate between the commercial and public sectors, is whether those actually charged with leading the NYPD change programme, were able to exert executive authority in the same way that one might expect to see it practised in the commercial setting. The question raised here is not intended to detract in any way from the immense improvements clearly made within the NYPD, but rather to question the extent to which the importance of maintaining a focus upon political capital implications, suggests that public service managers and leaders have to grapple with sensitivities that are not common in other sectors. For whilst environmental scanning and stakeholder awareness are key issues for all organisations, the requirement to maintain a positive out-turn in political capital terms is a unique challenge requiring a careful balance between the political and service imperatives – a role perhaps claimed by Weber-influenced bureaucrats.

The second key differentiator which it was suggested emerged from the NYPD case was the critical importance placed upon the achievement of appropriate metrics and having suitable levels of accountability attached to them. Whereas in the case of the political capital argument the view put forward was that this was an area of additional complexity largely alien to leaders in other sectors, the issue of measurement and performance focus is one where the public sector has been, to a great extent, behind other sectors in recognising their importance. That position has been largely challenged through the influential work of Giddens and other advocates of a 'third way' of politics adopted with enthusiasm by the Clinton administration in the USA and influential upon many other countries such as the UK, Australia and Canada (Giddens 1998). This 'third way' in essence revisits the doctrine of Thatcherism which, possibly to a far more lim-ited extent than is typically acknowledged, advocated that market dis-ciplines should be adopted within public service environments. The emergent models of practice that we see today in countries as geo-graphically separate as Australia, South Africa and the UK, are char-acterised by the high degree of prominence placed upon the achievement of targets, the attainment of pre-ordained service levels and the high degree of emphasis placed upon efficiency.

So can it be said that the 'we are different' argument is either much used or actually defensible in the modern world of leadership and management? An answer cannot hope to be comprehensive or defini-tive, for so much depends upon the context and perspective of the per-son attempting a response. The commonalties, as we have discussed in this section, are many and therefore suggest that there is a high degree of generic content to both the management and the leadership component associated with working within any organisation in the modern world. However, the key difference, that of the political dimension, is one which really may serve to set apart public service leadership style from that of other sectors. Added to this, the growing emphasis upon performance management and accountability within new models of public service also suggests that potentially even those who may have been adept at leading in a complex political environ-ment in the past, find themselves facing new challenges that are unfamiliar and potentially, in their articulation and deployment, lacking in the maturity and sensitivity to be wholly appropriate within the context that they are being deployed.

LEADING IN THE ABSENCE OF 'PROFIT'

Probably the one commonly understood 'differentiator' between the commercial and other sectors, is that the critical determinant of business success, bottom-line financial performance, as expressed in profit terms, has been held to be absent. The consequential impact of such a statement is potentially enormous. It suggests that what will result will be organisational cultures and behaviours that are not bottom-line focused and where, somehow, leadership style and personal motivation will echo a service ethic which is redolent with values from another era. Such a position requires careful consideration and a degree of constructive and informed challenge. It is arguable that what it does is to perpetuate yet another myth associated with the leadership of public service organisations: that leading in the absence of a requirement to show a financial profit must be the easier option.

The term 'profit' is one that is capable of many interpretations, but many definitions will include statements such as 'demonstrating a satisfactory return on investment'; 'maximising asset performance and returns'; and possibly even 'achieving objectives within resource constraints'. None of these, however, would appear to provide an automatic bar to the public service environment having a legitimate purchase, if so desired, on the term *profit*. Where perhaps we do move into unfamiliar territory, is when that part of the profit cycle concerned with balance-sheet performance and shareholder returns comes to the fore. For public services, these are areas that have, until very recently, been unfamiliar territory.

However, in the last five years there has been some considerable blurring of the lines, in some public service models at least, around the use and allied interpretations of the term 'profit'. The views put forward by Osborne and Gaebler, a decade ago, which urged that there was virtue in seeking to turn 'the profit motive to public use', are gaining wider adoption (Osborne and Gaebler 1992: 196). Quite whether the enthusiasm proffered by these authors has been translated into the innovative and inspirational practice that they suggest is possible, is questionable, however.

We may take as an example of the move towards an overt emphasis on profit and loss within the public services that of the United Kingdom's National Health Service (NHS). A service funded in entirety from revenues raised through general taxation, the organisation is huge and complex; to give some sense of its overall scope, it is the largest single employer in Europe and aims to provide comprehensive health-care literally from the cradle to the grave. As an organisation entering its sixth decade, its costs and allied complexities have soared, along with citizen expectations of a modern health service.

The NHS has been subject to many attempts at reform over the period of Thatcherism and beyond that, through to the impact of the

Blair government's intention to modernise service provision. Critically, for those charged with leading service delivery through a plethora of locally based trusts, a key plank of modernisation has been the requirement to manage services and service development within a negotiated and supposedly planned (over a three-year cycle) budget-setting process. Senior managers, particularly Chief Executives, are held accountable for their financial and service performance through the publication of an annual star rating. A key determinant of the rating achieved (these range from 0, the lowest, to 3, the very best), is that of financial performance – to deliver anything other than a balanced budget, is to gain an automatic zero rating. To gain a zero rating, as we shall discuss later in this chapter, is to invite unpalatable consequences for those leaders associated with it.

However, it is possible to argue that what is being delivered through this mechanism is an emphasis upon financial control rather than a genuine leveraging of the positive impacts of a profit motive. Analysis of policy development in this area does suggest, however, that what the NHS example points to is a linear progression, which sees a current focus upon the achievement of control. The next, and most contro-versial stage, is the creation of Foundation Hospitals, where the opportunities to trade, compete and raise money via commercial sector markets becomes possible for the first time with profit being fed back into growth and development. The opportunity to provide services with an intention to derive profit has incensed many politicians, leading to accusations that the public service ethos is being subverted with a resultant two-tier service emerging.

Setting aside overtly political debates, the critical question to raise here is whether current public service leaders are equipped to take control of such opportunities in effective and appropriate ways. Osborne and Gaebler, admittedly drawing their inspiration from small-scale pockets of innovation in the USA, advocated, even a decade ago, that modern public service leadership would be characterised by the need to be underpinned by entrepreneurial insight and confidence (Osborne and Gaebler 1992). For leaders within public services today the imperative to demonstrate entrepre-neurial behaviours is powerful – the capacity to demonstrate creative and 'out of the box' thinking, in respect of addressing key service challenges, is often a key tenet of senior-level person specifications.

Yet, what in practice does it actually mean to be profit-focused and entrepreneurial? Fundamentally, public services are predicated upon the requirement to serve citizens and other stakeholders – services and levels of provision are typically specified to a considerable level of detail. Where, within this recipe, can a leader find headroom and capacity to generate profit and to inspire an entrepreneurial culture throughout the organisation?

The example cited within the NHS has not yet been tested at a sufficient level of maturity to draw any generalisable conclusions. However, an organisation worthy of note, where there is considerable capacity for gaining insight into this critical area, is Centrelink; established over five years ago, it serves as the 'one-stop shop' for a wide range of Australian government services. Operating under the leadership of Sue Vardon, the Chief Executive, since its inception, Centrelink offers considerable opportunity for consideration of the extent to which focus upon financial control offers up the opportunity to innovate and grow the scope and remit of an organisation. Whilst the instinctive entrepreneurial tendencies exhibited by Vardon and the top team she has built around her have fed into the creation of a culture which appears to be both improvement- and opportunity-focused.

It is worth giving careful consideration to the lessons emerging from the Centrelink 'story':

'. . . It has evolved from a plan to integrate social security assistance and employment to a network of 1,000 sites of customer service centres, outreach services, agents and call centres providing a wide range of services on behalf of eleven Commonwealth (central government) and eleven state authorities. It employs 22,000 people and has 6 million customers spread the length and breadth of Australia. In the course of the evolution there have been many changes to the way service offerings are tailored.

In the creation of Centrelink, the Commonwealth Government set some simple and clear objectives:

■ Remove the complexity of government programmes for the customer
■ Create a one-stop shop for citizens
■ Introduce these services in the most efficient way, thereby providing savings to the government and the taxpayer
■ Maintain a high degree of accountability to government and hence the general public.'

(Milner 2002: 39)

As described above there can be little doubt that Centrelink represented, in its creation, an ambitious aspiration to create an organisation that was both performance- and service enhancement-focused. However, a constant 'bubble' above the heads of Vardon and other colleagues tasked with leading this major development, was the frequent reminder that they received from senior politicians that focus on a 'bottom line' was essential. Costs of service transactions had to be driven down whilst at the same time increasing service performance, in leadership and management terms, challenges familiar across many sectors. The 'carrot' held out for success in these areas was the potential to grow the scope and remit of Centrelink, the 'stick', the assurance that the government had no aversion to handing these areas of activity over to private sector providers.

The approach taken by Vardon, articulated in this case study in her own words, tells us much about the capacity of a public service leader to interpret profit creatively and to excite entrepreneurial instincts across a large and complex organisation.

'Centrelink was built from two networks of the Department of Social Security and parts of the Department of Employment, Education, Training and Youth Affairs. Each had been in existence for decades and had developed quite different cultures. The social security culture was process based and controlled by tight rule of necessity to ensure that people received their correct entitlements and no more. They had introduced a customer service focus but the delivery of a payment was an end in itself for most people. Staff from Employment, Education and Youth Affairs were outcome focused. Job seekers were to be found work and students helped into an education opportunity. They were supported by guidelines and programme funds that gave a fair degree of creative opportunity for staff to tailor a solution according to the circumstances. Both groups of staff were strongly influenced at a personal level to come to work to make a difference and to "help people".

Those of us who were building Centrelink wanted to capture the best of both these cultures and at the same time to set a special identity for the new agency. We identified those characteristics which would define our place and purpose. We created our own shared behaviours – listening, respecting, finding solutions, behaving with integrity and exploring. From the beginning we were mindful that the ministers wanted better experiences for the citizen with government so we made customer focus a prime focus for our reforms . . .

A campaign of listening to customers started immediately. In the first 2 years we listened to around 9,500 customers in small, specific feedback workshops with Centrelink staff . . . We learned that customers do not care which departments had responsibility for providing for their needs; they did not care what the products were called; few knew the differences between the three tiers of government. They did care though about being able to tell their circumstances only once and being dealt with by a caring person. They wanted simplicity, accuracy and friendly service. These standards became our benchmarks for service improvement . . .

The look and feel of Centrelink offices started to change dramatically. Out went the forbidding counters to be replaced by brightly coloured, open-plan offices and plants. Many more points of service for interviews were opened by bringing the back office people forward to the frontline . . . Service by appointment started and customer liaison officers walked the queues to help people who only wanted information or to hand in a form. Queue management became a priority and length of time people waited was reduced in most places. Customer service training was introduced and customer service champions were trained. Name tags for all staff including the Chief Executive officer were required to be worn . . .

As Centrelink opened, so did its opportunities. The government had a face and a network throughout Australia to which it could attach further services. We took stock of our capabilities. These included expertise in high volumes of payments; a network outreaching to the whole of Australia; a customer service approach; call centres, a capacity to implement major policy change fairly rapidly and connection to local communities . . .

However, whilst Centrelink has been chosen as the preferred supplier for the social security system and the gateway to reform in employment, the rest of its work [Vardon is able to cite many other activities added since start-up] is based upon competitive tendering or presentation of a business case to bid for new business. We had to develop business acumen to understand our costs and to understand how to run a business, rather than a traditional bureaucracy. The staff of Centrelink constantly present us with ideas for new business offerings.'

(Milner 2002: 42–7)

The story of Centrelink, and the themes that Vardon highlights as being critical to moving it from start-up to successful embedding, sustained nurturing and maturing, represents an important one in respect of understanding what is meant, in the modern world, by leadership in the absence of a profit motive. For what we have seen here is an organisation which is unquestionably large, undoubtedly complex, being shaped to address shifting 'futures'. The time that Vardon prioritised at the outset, in setting out what Centrelink's culture and behaviours should be, provided an architecture, whereby the organisation has demonstrated itself to be capable of evolution and of adaptability in a competitive environment. Centrelink's instincts are unquestionably service-orientated but, critically too, they display key aspects of an entrepreneurial organisation – the desire to grow, the capacity to innovate and the creativity necessary to bring these about. Centrelink may not operate in the profit-obsessed commercial sector but it does inhabit a territory that public services have to increasingly populate, one where focus on the bottom line, married with innovation, represent the keys not only to success but also, potentially, to survival.

PERFORMANCE AND CONFORMANCE – CARROTS AND STICKS . . .

'You can't expect the government to just hope . . .' is a view expressed by the chairman of a newly created UK audit and inspection organisation, the Commission for Healthcare Audit and Inspection (CHAI) (Donnelly 2003: 22). In an era where globally there has been a significant challenge to the concept of 'big' and potentially unaccountable public services, the view expressed by Kennedy echoes the sentiments underpinning policy development in locations as geographically apart as Australia and Europe. 'Hope' is no longer sufficient, nor indeed it would appear are articulations of policy and strategy, the emphasis in the early part of the 21st century sits in the area of target-setting and performance metrics. For public service leaders the trend towards service delivery based around pre-ordained targets has touched almost every sector; within the UK, for example, bodies exist to monitor and report upon performance in a wide range of sectors, from education through to diverse aspects of local government delivery, not forgetting the largest single undertaking – that of health. One of these bodies, the Audit Commission, felt that such was the misunderstanding and, in their view, inappropriate criticism of the development of targets that they set out a formal response in a briefing report:

'It is widely recognised that government has a legitimate right to set national aspirations for improvement. There is also a shared appreciation that performance indicators are crucial in reporting progress, telling a rounded story about performance and enabling comparisons and learning between services and organisations. It is the effectiveness of nationally set targets that is central to the criticisms. These criticisms have challenged the number of targets, who sets them, and the interaction between setter and user.

This does not mean that targets should be dismissed. Targets are invaluable when used well and as one part of a robust performance management framework. They can align user expectations and service priorities and, in doing so, motivate frontline staff.

This alignment should not always be viewed as a simple cascade from national government to local deliverers. The focus on "localism" and tailoring services to the needs of individuals and diverse groups has created a different context within which public services are being delivered and targets are being used. In addition, there is an increasing emphasis on complex quality of life improvements in localities which can only be delivered through partnerships.

These forces demand change – a rebalancing from nationally set targets to targets set by local organisations. A change that should make targets more intelligent, grounded in what works, and recognises the influence of contextual factors.

Nationally set targets are still required. They are powerful in providing a focus on the experience of service users. For them to work there are a number of factors that need to be present: user expectations should be similar across the country; there should be wide knowledge of what works; and accountability for improvement should primarily be national. When these factors are absent, the target setting is best left to localities. However, diversity of performance and a lack of trust suggest the pace and extent of this shift will be different for different organisations. Ultimately, intelligent target setting needs a dialogue between government and individual localities.

In summary, targets are invaluable and here to stay . . .'

(Audit Commission 2003: 1)

With such certainty emerging around the environment in which public services will have to operate in the coming decades some key questions arise around the scope for displaying leadership in a climate where success or otherwise is defined by conformance to externally set targets. Central to this area are questions raised by Ian Kennedy, the incoming chairman of CHAI:

'I've made it fairly clear that I think we should be concerned with monitoring and inspecting against standards, but with a view to seeking to help and share best practice ... A plethora of targets seems to me to get in the way of allowing professionals to get on with what we pay them to use – namely their profession and their judgement ... While the government has an entitlement to say what, globally, should be delivered by the NHS, the bodies it sets up, such as CHAI, must be able to negotiate if they think that targets are distorting the delivery of services.'

(Donnelly 2003: 23)

One of the concerns of this book is to look at leadership for adaptive change under a performance management regime such as that pioneered in the United Kingdom, where published league tables for schools and star ratings for hospitals and general practice are now the established norm. There are tensions in this situation that fundamentally steer us towards wondering how a necessary perspective on the value of national targets and the achievement of conformance in respect of them can be combined effectively with innovative and entrepreneurial leadership styles. If the tension between conformance to national targets and standards and entrepreneurial leadership cannot be handled constructively there is a danger of inhibiting leadership. For example, a pessimistic view would predict that a 21st century UK public service leader might share some common characteristics such as:

- sense of disconnection from ownership of an improvement agenda
- perception that the external and nationally focused targets override and overwhelm local priorities
- occupation of a shared common 'space' where blame is the key driver and failure is an unacceptable option – clearly such an environment must serve to impact on both the confidence and commitment of key individuals.

What has been considered above is obviously an extremely pessimistic view of the effects of a performance agenda that is widespread in public services. As we noted in the case study of the New York City Police Department, performance analysis is treated as a key improvement tool with regular opportunities for testing data and those responsible for it. However, the role of performance within the NYPD can be characterised as representing part of a continuum, where the goals and objectives are clearly stated, with the scope for local intervention and leadership clearly enshrined in the organisational development model. The cases we look at in Chapter 6 also show how public service leaders have successfully combined vision, strategy and performance management. Nevertheless, there is a danger in the modernising agenda all around the world, including the UK, that the performance process becomes all-pervading to the detriment of entrepreneurial leadership at all levels of the public service. Then it would be inextricably linked to a sense of sole outcome – that you either conform or that you do not.

Whilst of course, no one could subscribe to the notion of a public service leader, responsible for a failing organisation, avoiding all possible sanctions, the notion of building into a performance-orientated model a capacity, as Kennedy has stressed, for 'learning', is an important one (Donnelly 2003: 23). If, fundamentally, the adoption of key performance indicators, metrics and targets, is to build public confidence and instil in public services some of the key disciplines found in the commercial sector, then it is important that leaders in public services feel confident that such an approach is process-focused, incremental and capable of local interpretation.

If we return to the example of Centrelink considered earlier in this chapter, clearly the view set out by the CEO, Sue Vardon, was that the organisation's very survival was predicated upon a need to demonstrate reduced operating costs whilst attaining increased user satisfaction. To attain this ambitious position, and indeed to sustain it, required, as we explored previously, high degrees of inspirational and behaviour-setting leadership from the very top. However, Vardon argues, it required something profoundly different also:

'The biggest cultural shift for everyone was to become performance-focused as we were funded through business partnership agreements and had to satisfy regularly measured key performance indicators. A balanced score card was introduced to emphasise this performance-focused approach. The Kaplan and Norton model for developing such a scorecard approach was used. Key performance areas were determined for each of Centrelink's five corporate goals and an emphasis was placed upon achieving vertical integration of the scorecard throughout the organisation. Disparate performance data sources were brought together into one central assessment point and presented as green (met) and yellow (unmet) dots. Identifying and developing robust measurements which would serve to drive forward the goal of performance improvement, particularly in respect of defining metrics for those areas traditionally hard to capture into substantive data, took many months.'

(Milner 2002: 42)

Here we see a leadership model that operates within a high expectation performance culture – but critically, it is one where leaders within that organisation have been trusted to take forward a performance agenda. Centrelink and the NYPD both represent high-achieving, globally acknowledged success stories associated with substantial improvements in service performance. If we contrast this with a conformance- and target-focused approach to the development of public services, such as that extant in the United Kingdom, it is possible to argue that the conformance model so limits the opportunities for local leadership, that the profound cultural change that the Australian and US case studies have alluded to, is all but impossible to achieve.

So where and how can leadership flourish in public service cultures that are characterised by an emphasis upon the need to meet and improve upon performance issues on an ongoing basis? Where there is an extreme interpretation of the role of performance, in essence where the emphasis upon conformance dominates and potentially distorts all other organisational priorities, one has to question the potential for leadership traits to actually develop or be demonstrated effectively. The conformance model is one that sees all leadership figures potentially giving all of their energies to the achievement of externally set targets. To deliver upon this type of management model requires, of itself, high degrees of resilience and compliance focus and it is questionable whether such an approach is sustainable over the longer term.

A further perspective upon leadership in a regulated and performance-driven public service culture, is one which is equally demanding, but potentially altogether more positive, that of performance management representing part of an integrated whole. In this articulation of the potential for leadership to make a demonstrable difference, performance issues are just as centrally located as they are within the conformance model, it is the scope for local ownership which represents the key difference. In Chapter 6 we will see that some public services leaders work hard to build this ownership of the performance figures among managers and staff, and although this is not easy to do it is a responsibility of leadership in a democratically accountable public service. But there is also an issue here about the elected politicians creating the conditions in which there is scope for organisational leadership and ownership of performance in relation to the public's needs. Organisational leaders need the space to set performance indicators that underpin their assessment of the needs of their public. This not only applies to the case of local government, where organisationally specific performance indicators are needed to reflect local diversity. As Vardon recalls, Centrelink's process of locally owned consultation with citizens was enlightening:

'The staff who were listening were surprised by some of the feedback and often made immediate improvements to their local office. On one occasion the feedback was that the sign saying "We reserve the right to call the police if your behaviour is offensive" made them feel like criminals. The sign had been placed up to warn a few people but the effect had been generalised . . . The look and feel of Centrelink offices began to change dramatically. Out went forbidding counters to be replaced by brightly coloured, open-plan offices and plants. Many more points of service for interviews were opened by bringing the back office people forward to the frontline . . . Queue management became a priority and the length of time people waited was reduced in most places.'

(Milner 2002: 45)

CHAPTER 4

THE LEADERSHIP TRAJECTORY

In Chapter 3 we discussed the fact that a focus upon leadership could be located within a wider trajectory that can be observed in management theory and practice over a period of more than two decades. Leadership represents, if you like, a point in the organisational change and development cycle that moves to prominence when many others have been trialled and have delivered limited but important returns. For public services the drive towards quality management and service improvement and redesign has mirrored much of what can be observed occurring in other sectors from the early 1980s onwards. The thought that 'if you can't measure it, you can't manage it' is a blunt instrument perhaps, but one which permeates a good deal of public service thinking to this very day. However, it is arguable that such a focus, if pursued excessively, will stifle the potential of organisations to do anything more than seek to conform. The type and style of leadership associated with such overtly operational achievement cultures can be so outcome- and conformance-focused that their credibility and resilience can be sustained over only limited life-cycles.

If an increasing focus upon leadership points to one element that public service organisations are increasingly realising is critical to ongoing success and improvement, it is to the issue of sustainability. Conformance cultures can only be sustained for relatively short periods before human nature and resistance to overt controls comes into play. Sustaining improvements in performance over the longer term requires an altogether more sophisticated approach to the service model and to the role of leadership within it. For as we have seen in the examples of Centrelink and the NYPD the service model is based upon an approach to performance improvement which unquestionably places these issues centre stage. However, the critical differentiator in analysing such organisations which might be categorised as demonstrating high degrees of maturity, is undoubtedly the extent to which the performance agenda is owned by the organisation rather than being centrally imposed. In organisations such as this, leadership and performance issues are inextricably intertwined because they represent a shared agenda where conformance naturally occurs because the key leadership behaviours and messages resonate with a passion for, and commitment to, performance improvement. Nurturing and enabling such cultures, it might be argued, is far more likely to provide governments with assurance that they can do much more than 'hope' that improvement and service change will occur.

WHO ARE THE LEADERS? THE ROLE OF POLITICS IN PUBLIC SERVICE LEADERSHIP

Public service leaders are employed within organisational contexts such that they need to demonstrate a capacity to both inhabit and navigate a way through overtly political territory. This factor alone represents the key leadership difference between the public service environment and that of other sectors. Public services, their vision, values and direction, are owned only in part by those charged with moving the organisation forward. Politicians, who in democratic models of society are subject to the exigency of demonstrating close awareness of election life-cycles, can be prone to the adoption of short-termist and populist-focused agenda. Reflecting upon and perhaps deflecting this view of the drivers of public service, James Callaghan, former Prime Minister of the United Kingdom, pondered when asked whether politicians worried too much about the short term, about opinion polls and the next election:

'It is a problem of course, because people want to win the next election and the closer you get to an election the more your supporters in Parliament or in Congress want to keep their seats. Successful leaders, however, do become a little removed from short-term considerations.

You cannot sit in the Prime Minister's chair at Number Ten Downing Street without feeling that you are a trustee both of the past and of the future. That sense of obligation, perhaps, does make life a little difficult when you have five year parliamentary elections.'

(Webber 1986: 110)

A key question to ask when considering the potential for a leadership dichotomy in public services is whether the capacity or 'space' actually exists for political and managerial service leaders to co-exist. This potential tension arises out of the bureaucratic legacies of government and public services more generally which have operated upon a presumption that there could be a relatively neat division of policy leadership (held by the politicians) and managerial implementation (the role of the service employees and managers).

If we consider the importance of understanding why politicians may have inherently felt more comfortable when working on the premise that they alone were the leaders and that public service personnel were managers, Zaleznik's influential work of some three decades ago provides useful perspective:

'Managers tend to adopt impersonal, if not passive, attitudes toward the goals . . . whereas leaders adopt a personal and active attitude toward them.

Managers tend to view work as an enabling process involving some combination of people and ideas interacting to establish strategies and make decisions.

Leaders work from high-risk positions, indeed often are temperamentally disposed to seek out risk and danger, especially where opportunity and reward appear high.

Managers prefer to work with people; they avoid solitary activity because it makes them anxious. They relate to people according to the role they play in a sequence of events or in a decision-making process, while leaders are concerned with ideas, relate in more intuitive and empathetic ways.'

(Zaleznik 1977: 23)

Acceptance that leadership wherever it is positioned requires pro-activity, confidence and creativity immediately sets up a potential tension within a highly directional model of political policy-setting. To return to the Centrelink example it is possible in retrospect to plot the policy articulation through to service design and delivery and to consider the capacity that this model has allowed for leadership within the organisation to be nurtured for service benefit. To take first the policy articulation set out by the Australian Prime Minister in 1997:

'From the moment I entered Parliament in 1974 and began talking to constituents about their various problems, I began hearing complaints about the number of agencies you had to visit. And what focused my mind at the time was that so many people felt that if only they could go to one place and have all their business done in that one spot it would be a lot more efficient, it would be a lot more human and it would make a great deal more sense. The consolidation in Centrelink of so many of the services of the government that interact with people will provide, of course, a more human face and a more efficient service. In the past we have encouraged people to go from one location to another and we have often confused them with a lot of administrative duplication. And in one very big stroke Centrelink cuts through that duplication. Centrelink consolidates in an efficient modern fashion the major service delivery activities of the federal government.'

(Milner 2002: 40–1)

If we set alongside this the views set out by the United Kingdom's Prime Minister, Tony Blair, in respect of aspirations for the NHS:

'Our challenge is to modernise government and raise the quality and accessibility of all our public services. We acknowledge that people leading busy working lives should not be obliged to queue up during the working day to get to the services they are entitled to. They should be able to access services how and when they want. There are some first rate services . . . like NHS Direct, or NHS Walk-in Centres, which show the way forward. We need to build on these examples.

The first rate public services of tomorrow will respond quickly to the needs and wishes of its users and produce innovative solutions to the problems that emerge.'

(Cabinet Office 2001: 1)

For both of these eminent politicians the policy agenda is clear and they articulate a powerful vision of reform-focused service delivery. However, analysis of the practice and potential for leadership that underpins the political dimension provides key indicators as to the complex dimensions that exist when seeking to occupy a leadership role within a politically driven environment. Within this book we have given close attention to the Centrelink model, particularly because it exemplifies a productive engagement between the politically driven policy agenda and the capacity for creative organisational development to emerge, under CEO and team leadership which whilst embedded in, and mirroring the policy objectives, has had the confidence to take forward a challenging agenda. Within Centrelink the role of leadership, at all levels of the organisation, as a critical success factor is particularly strong. However, it may be that this case study represents an all too rare balance between the political and the service delivery dynamic.

To return to Tony Blair's articulation of a vision for the National Health Service (NHS), such sentiments are very much in alignment with those presented by John Howard. The policy drivers around citizen-centric service delivery are almost identical. The challenge is how to stimulate the potential for service-based leadership in line with the policy dimension. As was discussed in the previous chapter, the application of performance- and conformance-driven targets and indicators is common across public services. However, the danger is that the innovation agenda becomes stifled by a conformance culture. There is also danger from a conformance culture if the political drive to use organisational audits as an instrument of reform is not linked to a proper understanding of recent service experience and results. It is critical that empirical experience teaches what works and what does not work. In measured and tempered tones the Audit Commission posits a view that the UK system of auditing using star ratings is 'only weakly related to performance or management ability' (Audit Commission 2003).

Research around the key characteristics of public service, and particularly health care leadership, led by Professor Andrew Pettigrew, provides some interesting insights into the way in which the political and strategic dimensions of leadership need to be understood and tested. Pettigrew's thesis appears to be built around a central questioning of whether leadership by executives of public service organisations can actually make a difference to the likely success or otherwise of a public service organisation. Key themes arising out of his work provide an apparently guarded answer of 'yes' to such a question, but only in situations where the degree of political micro-management did not serve to render impotent the ability of service employees to lead. Summarising Pettigrew's key behaviours associated with successful public service leaders we see an emphasis upon the following:

- a willingness to experiment;
- an ability to develop and communicate clear organisational objectives and how they are to be achieved;
- the ability to manage the process of organisational change and to customise it to fit local conditions;
- a demonstrable ability to foster good relationships with stakeholders and partners within the wider community;
- a willingness to use performance measurement and management techniques to help drive change;
- a recognition that good performance is multi-dimensional.

(www.nhsconfed.net 2001)

Views such as these are important in as much as they set out the expectations associated with holding a public service leadership role in the 21st century. They are also, viewed in one dimension, entirely reasonable and demonstrably capable of being delivered upon if we consider cases referred to in this book such as Centrelink, the NYPD, and the UK examples in Chapter 6. However, as these cases also demonstrate, there is an issue about the political skills of managerial leaders and how they manage their relationship with elected politicians. It has also to be said that the prevailing view in a number of countries that politicians do politics and managers do management is not helpful in this regard. The managerial leaders of the public services are in political roles and have to have political skills but they are not able to use a legitimate language of political management to discuss and explore the issues they face. This denial of a legitimate language appropriate to their de facto role in politics places them at a disadvantage in asking the right questions and seeking appropriate answers. But when this is all said and done, there is a major responsibility on elected politicians to enable managers to provide leadership in the 21st century. For leaders to be willing themselves to take risks, for example, there must be a reasonable degree of trust in their political counterparts that if failure or only partial achievement were to result, that the responsibility whilst accepted by those in positions of leadership would not automatically be punitive in nature.

In considering the role of the politician and of the political dimension within the public service environment, it is important also to consider the impact that these factors have upon this sector to recruit and retain the very best current and future leaders. With public services internationally having an aspiration to transform and to become not only more effective but also visibly more citizen-focused, the requirement to attract to, and retain within, the sector the very best talent represents an ongoing matter of concern. Setting aside the observation that for some decades now the public service environment has been steadily losing out in the 'hiring' game to the more attractive and apparently dynamic sectors such as finance and technology, we see instead a real paucity of talent apparently being willing, albeit that the salary rewards and packages have typically outpaced inflation, to take on emergent leadership challenges. The reasons for much of this sit outside the direct remit of this work, yet certainly an issue which sits squarely within the boundaries of leadership, is that of actually having, particularly at the most senior levels, a clear mandate to lead. Where there is leadership 'haze' and politicians are seen to be actually neutralising the ability of even the most talented executives to do anything other than work towards the achievement of targets, then the relative attractiveness of the public sector diminishes still further.

Whilst in many countries government departments are actively setting up leadership colleges and allied programmes, it is perhaps worth asking, where do politicians learn about their role in the political leadership of public service organisations? Politicians typically adopt situational leadership styles; they begin by articulating policy that mirrors a political position and then adapt it as they assess the likelihood of political gains accruing from its implementation. As we suggest in Chapter 6, the politicians approach radical change, therefore, ideologically. They are dependent on the managerial leaders to supply the necessary organisational expertise they lack. If they fail to work with the managerial leaders in this way, their adaptive and politically driven style actually serves to diminish leadership credibility and the confidence of managers and staff in the reform process – thus actually serving to limit the potential for policy success to accrue.

Gerald Ford, perhaps best remembered as being an 'accidental' president of the United States, reflected upon the role of the politicians and how they should, he believed, interact with those of the service leaders:

'As a new (political) leader, you must be perceived as totally honest, dedicated to the proper goals, and possessed of the strength necessary to achieve results. Everyone must see you as a person of integrity – people on the inside with whom you work as well as people outside . . .. Everyone must understand that you take action only to pull things together, that you will act in the best interests of all concerned . . .. As a new president, I had to instil a feeling within the government that I was working to get things back on an even keel . . . Parallels exist, of course, between the circumstances I inherited and those in corporations where previous management has been challenged for mismanagement or corruption . . .. Fundamentally though you delegate to people the responsibility for running their own operations. You give them a firm outline of their duties, then hold them responsible.'

(Webber 1987: 77–8)

A valuable additional perspective on this position is articulated by Mary Harney, Deputy Prime Minister of the Republic of Ireland, a country internationally recognised for both its economic success and its public service reform strategy:

> 'The key is to have a policy-making system that is sufficiently flexible to respond to changing circumstances, but is sufficiently consistent in relation to its core policies to ensure that uncertainty in relation to the stance of future governments is minimised. Implementing this on a national level requires a high degree of awareness on the part of government, an ability to communicate with the citizens of the country and a shared commitment to achieve objectives.'
>
> (Milner 2002: 155)

It is possible to argue that at the time of writing, the relationship between the political leadership and managerial leadership of public services has never been more in need of development. It is not an issue of clear boundaries between politicians and managers. It is about both elected politicians and managerial leaders learning to combine for effective political management and leadership of services. The boundaries between the roles have become blurred and require managerial leaders to develop political skills. For those concerned with the study of leadership this represents a key concern and indeed potential barrier to the achievement of more wholesale changes in the way in which public services are designed and delivered. The challenges of public service leadership in the strategic and operational contexts are huge and require that the very best talent should be deployed into leading and developing a momentum for real and sustained change. However, where the public service environment has gained a reputation for being characterised by political micro-management and poor political skills among top managers, then clearly the leadership role is going to look as though only very exceptional people can survive in it. The lessons in leadership that are discussed here would, upon this analysis, point to a further dimension that requires a focus upon development, that being the imperative to inculcate appropriate leadership styles and behaviours amongst those operating in the overtly political domain.

FOLLOWERSHIP

Almost regardless of sector, close engagement with the considerable literature located around matters of leadership can leave one with the impression that for an organisation to be successful, all it requires is good, or ideally great, leadership. However, what such discussions typically fail to explore, is the essentially symbiotic relationship between an organisation's leadership capacity and its innate ability to be led. Establishing an organisational culture, which is receptive to being led, has often been the first critical test of senior personnel upon taking up their post. In public services this can be particularly so, if we return once more to the notion of the bureaucratic model which was entrenched over many decades. If we consider the forces of change and modernisation which have been deployed across the public service globe and which have dismantled the service model that was so beloved of generations of 'public servants' or 'government officers', then it is relevant to ask, how do people learn the capacity to respond to the new challenges of being led?

Under the public service reform agenda pioneered by the administrations of Margaret Thatcher and Ronald Reagan, new service models were developed which sought to import some of the disciplines of the commercial sector. Service level agreements and the internal market began to change the ways in which employees of public service organisations related to one another. Yet fundamentally, in retrospect, such developments, whilst representing a critical point in the life-cycle of public services, did little to actually impact on the numbers employed in public services, nor the fundamentally silo-based ways of working that had grown up under the bureaucratic tradition. At this point in the 1980s it was possible to argue that public services were far less exercised by the need for leadership and were rather more concerned with the necessity to import and adopt management practices from other sectors.

Within the evolutionary cycle of public service change it is possible to plot the first energising reforms as being predicated upon a belief that improved management techniques and abilities would be the keys to transformation (see Chapter 1). However, the reform journey has proved to be a long and challenging one and after some two decades of change, it is possible to observe that the emphasis has now shifted to the need for leadership. However, underpinning all of this, is that structurally, and perhaps even philosophically, public services today retain elements of unwieldiness and strict adherence to practices and boundaries which render them challenging environments to reform. Where leaders seek to challenge established practices, it is wise to make no assumptions that those employed within the organisation will automatically follow, nor should the capacity for wide-scale cynicism and subversion of a change agenda, no matter how compellingly communicated, be underestimated.

The inextricable relationship between that of leading and following has long been debated within the military sphere and it is worthy of note here, when one considers that so much of the bureaucratic traditions of public service have been modelled upon the military context. Historians advocate that Napoleon is one of the best examples of leadership that can be translated, from both negative and positive perspectives, into the modern organisational context. It is certainly worth noting as Kim *et al.* suggest that Napoleon's early leadership behaviour gives good insight as to how to inspire a culture of 'followership':

'If we look at Napoleon's early battles, his relationship with his men was defined by openness, close interaction and exchange. He used "fair process" in the formulation and execution of his strategies and tactics ... Napoleon would prove a master at getting the most out of his men despite limited resources and no reputation ... Napoleon believed in making the simplest soldier a party to his plans and spelling out what was demanded. He treated soldiers with enormous respect for the importance of their contribution. On the eve of the battle of Austerlitz in 1805, Napoleon famously rode over 30 miles up and down his ranks, tiring out horses and staff while informing his troops of the next day's battle plan ... it was the first time in history that a leader had revealed his plan to the entire army. Bonaparte knew of his men's needs and motivation and how critical their commitment was to victory at Austerlitz. Taking his men into his confidence raised their morale, provided them with a clear plan and literally won half the battle before it began . . .. He understood the advantages of engaging his officers and liked to explain and discuss his strategic plans with them, seeking their reactions and advice.'

(Kim *et al.* 2002: 5)

So, at the outset at least, the leadership style exemplified here was one which the modern-day leadership commentator could generally empathise with. Here is a leader who is results-orientated, can communicate and contextualise a clear vision and goals whilst inspiring a willingness to engage, contribute and follow in those at all levels subordinate to him.

However, Napoleon whilst capable of providing a powerful example of transformational leadership from which many generalisable lessons can be extracted, did not mature into a still greater leader. Instead, success diminished his leadership traits, such that the once inclusive and empowering leader became someone who would no longer:

'. . . deal with his generals directly, communicating orders, promotions, sackings and the like through his newly appointed chief of staff. But at the same time he refused to allow anyone to make the smallest decision without his stamp of approval. Many of his close followers were no longer on speaking terms and most were distrustful of one another. All were wary of their leader.'

(Kim *et al.* 2002: 5)

Such extremes of leadership paradigm as exemplified by one individual give us powerful insight into the role of the leader and the consequential relationship that style and behaviour has upon the extent to which 'followership' is gained. Kim, in his analysis of Napoleon at his most charismatic, empowering and endearing, signalled that one of the greatest strengths that Napoleon exemplified at this stage in his career, was his instinctive adherence to the concept of 'fair process'. Such a concept is critical to our understanding of how, within the public service domain, a leader may seek to leverage the likelihood of being ultimately successful. As Kim explains:

'In practical terms, fair process encapsulates three mutually reinforcing principles: engagement, explanation and clarity of expectations. Engagement means involving people in the decisions that affect them by asking for their input and allowing them to argue the merits of one another's ideas and assumptions . . .. The second principle involves explaining the reasons for decisions to all involved parties . . .. Clarity of expectations requires that once a decision is made, the new rules of the game are clearly stated. . .. When fair process is exercised in decision-making, individuals are inspired to go beyond the call of duty in sharing their ideas and voluntarily co-operating. But when fair process is violated, co-operation and the sharing of knowledge suffer and people exercise retributive justice to make amends for the improper treatment they receive. This can include shirking, sabotaging efforts and withholding co-operation.'

(Kim *et al.* 2002: 5)

The 'fair process' view of leadership would appear to be one which is particularly apposite for those with an interest in developing models of leadership which are likely to be successful in the public service environment. Focusing upon the need to engage with, and gain sign-up from, key allies and indeed colleagues at all levels of an organisation, is a theme which has particular resonance when scanning examples of public service leadership at both extremes of the Napoleon paradigm. Critical to success in public service reform and development is acknowledgement that profound change requires not only champions, it requires willing actors who will follow a lead. Kim's insight is a particularly useful one to feed into this discussion of the importance of leaders being able to create an environment where following is both acceptable and motivating:

'In our decade-long research into leadership, we found that a critical but frequently forgotten dimension is the process by which a leader interacts with his or her people to make decisions. Our systematic research shows the causal relationship between procedural fairness and the quality and execution of strategic directions . . .. Fair process may have been largely ignored in leadership, but we found that this dimension could make or break a leader.'

(Kim and Mauborgne 2003: 26)

LEADING CHANGE AND RENEWAL – THE ULTIMATE ASPIRATION FOR PUBLIC SERVICE?

Modern public services exist within operating environments where typically one of the few certainties is the articulation at a policy level of the need for change and improvement. The emphasis upon change has become almost as embedded within this sector as it has in more commercially orientated environments. It is likely that the current 'obsession' with leadership as a generic trait within the public service environment stems almost entirely from a perception that successful change requires a certain type of leadership. The subliminal message being that public services have not been as adept at changing and developing as they might have been because they do not benefit from the 'right types' of leadership. However, caution must be exerted here, for the very concept of change is often interpreted as a blunt instrument, it is something which is 'done to' organisations. Kanter suggests a rather more tempered view:

> 'Certain kinds of change appear to come easily – bold strokes by leaders that turn the world upside down . . .. But transforming the way an organization operates and how its people work is a long march, requiring many individuals to change their behaviour over a long period of time. Change is full of false starts, messy mistakes, and controversial experiments involving the participation and guidance of many people. Even bold strokes are merely announcements of intention whose success will depend on the longer march to implementation. It is tempting for leaders to try to transform their organization by throwing everything out and starting over again, but it is more effective to nurture changes already developing within the organization.'
>
> (Kanter 1997: 65)

Kanter's view is a realistic one; it notes the need for change to be an involving process and one that is allowed to mature over time. It invites one to see change processes as part of a wider continuum where, over time, the organisation has not simply undergone a change process, it has demonstrated the capacity to *renew* itself. The term 'renewal' is an important one within the context of the public service arena, for the close connotations that it bears to the spiritual and overtly service dimensions of organisational capacity, often represent the missing elements from a formal change process. Organisations, which are seeking to renew typically, have a clear underlying purpose and mission – what might often be referred to as the 'public service ethic'. However, they acknowledge that, as structured and focused, they are limited in their capacity to develop in ways which are appropriate. Organisations considered within this book where one might usefully point to renewal being an unspoken aspiration, are clearly the NYPD and Centrelink. In both cases complex public service 'tasks' have been considered in ways that are considerably more appropriate for the times we inhabit. Service offerings have been developed which reflect the need to refocus, whilst at the same time there is clear evidence of the importance placed by leaders upon renewing and strengthening the bonds of public service commitment.

Leading renewal can never be a 'quick fix' strategy, as Kanter argues such approaches are:

> '. . . led by people who are comfortable with ambiguity. Leaders of change are willing to commit to long-term goals and to persist in achieving them, they are participative and inclusive in their management styles. They bring skills to every stage of the change drama. In the first phase they translate vague assignments into projects by tuning in to their environment, challenging assumptions and crafting a vision. Next, using diplomatic skills to get favorable responses, they build coalitions of backers and supporters willing to invest in the effort and to help it over the hurdles. . .'
>
> (Kanter 1997: 67)

Successful public service development and the concept of 'quick fixes' do not typically sit comfortably alongside one another. As we have discussed, leadership is critical within this sector, just as much as in any other, if sustainable and appropriate change is to be achieved. However, it is important not to underestimate the high levels of complexity involved in making any attempt to lead a public service organisation towards a point not only of change but also of ongoing capacity for renewal. Through our discussions we have clearly set out a view that there are some key factors which clearly do differentiate the challenges of leading in this sector from those of others. However, they do not render the challenges impossible; that leadership and renewal are possible we have already seen and will continue to explore in the following chapters.

CHAPTER 5

DEFINING PUBLIC SERVICES LEADERSHIP

LEADERS AND NEW PUBLIC MANAGEMENT

Any discussion of a concept as potentially nebulous as that of 'leadership' requires that some articulation of a definition should be attempted. However, it is important that any emergent definition should be capable of reflecting, as Bennis suggests is essential, that leadership is a complex social phenomenon, lacking real boundaries and where a clear definition is likely to be elusive (Bennis 1959). A further element of complexity is added when one specifies still further, that it is leadership within a particular sector that is being considered. Extensive reviews of the literature can leave one with only a single certainty, that being that there is no single agreed definition of what leadership is, or indeed where within organisations it is principally located. Analysis of discussions over some three decades within the public services environment, leaves us also with some sense of confusion. Within the critical development of what is perhaps best termed the 'philosophy' of New Public Management (NPM) we find that there is a predominance of references to the need for 'management' and it is only latterly that leadership *per se* has become evident as a subject for critical review. Unpacking the variety of definitions in use and the apparent interchangeability of the terms *management* and *leadership* within the public service environment is thus a key challenge to address within this chapter.

We would like to return to the definition provided by Kotter (see Chapter 2) who both addresses what leadership may be and posits a view as to how it should be differentiated from the act of management:

'Leadership is different from management, but not for the reasons most people think. Leadership isn't mystical and mysterious. It has nothing to do with having "charisma" or other exotic personality traits. It is not the province of a chosen few. Nor is leadership necessarily better than management or a replacement for it.

Rather leadership and management are two distinctive and complementary systems of action. Each has its own function and characteristic activities. Both are necessary for success in [today's] . . . environment.

Management is about coping with complexity. Its practices and procedures are largely a response to . . . the emergence of large complex organizations . . . Leadership, by contrast, is about coping with change. Part of the reason it has become so important in recent years is that the . . . world has become more competitive and more volatile. . . . More change always demands more leadership.'

(Kotter 1990: 72)

Kotter's exposition of a rationale, in the modern organisation, for understanding the differences between management and leadership represents one of the most influential starting-points in seeking to define, within a public service environment, what leadership can, and indeed does, represent. In Chapter 6 we use recent case study evidence to question the completeness of his definition or the appropriateness of his definition for public services leadership. Nevertheless, the themes that Kotter highlights, whilst addressed primarily to a commercial sector audience, have considerable relevance and resonance for those engaged in seeking to transform public services. By allying the concept of leadership to that of organisational change, a sense of embedding in real processes is fostered; leadership ceases to be a somewhat nebulous and remote 'quality' and instead becomes a key component of any attempts to reform or transform an organisation.

Any focus upon leadership centred upon the public service domain requires that the political and indeed philosophical dimensions of the global reform agenda are taken into account. By doing so, it is possible to plot a developmental trajectory which saw, as the Organisation for Economic Co-operation and Development (OECD) highlighted in the mid-1990s, that: 'a new paradigm for public management has emerged, aimed at fostering a performance-oriented culture in a less centralized public sector' (OECD 1995: 8). This 'new paradigm' is often referred to as New Public Management and in itself the term refers rather more to a developmental journey than to an agreed set of principles. Building upon, or representing a corrective action to, many of the dominant themes of public service reform in the 1980s, which were typically characterised by the introduction of quasi-market disciplines and a challenge to bureaucratic traditions, NPM can be said to focus upon achieving qualitative service improvement, from a citizen perspective, whilst maintaining an overt focus upon bottom-line financial performance. From the early adopters of this stance, New Zealand and Canada, through to more recent advocates such as Germany, analysis of practice emphasises the symbiotic relationship between the implementation of change and the presence of leadership to carry forward a reform agenda.

The use of the word 'new' is instructive when considering the relationship between leadership and change within public services, for this perhaps more than any other area, points to areas of real change in philosophy and expectation. This builds upon and contextualises Osborne and McLaughlin's suggestion, that through their extensive reviews of literature and global practice, it is possible to argue that NPM is comprised of seven key 'doctrines':

- 'a focus on hands-on and entrepreneurial management as opposed to the traditional bureaucratic focus of the public administrator;
- explicit standards and measures of performance;
- an emphasis upon output controls;
- the importance of desegregation and decentralization of public services;
- a shift to the promotion of competition in the provision of public services;
- a stress on private sector styles of management and their superiority; and
- the promotion of discipline and parsimony in resource allocation.'
(McLaughlin *et al.* 2002: 9)

It is in the combination of these key points that we can begin to see the impact of NPM emerging globally, admittedly at different speeds and with great capacity for local interpretation being demonstrated. However, what is all too rarely focused upon are the leadership challenges faced by those charged with taking forward this complex change agenda. To seek to lead, as Kotter outlined at the beginning of this chapter, is to do something other than to manage, yet paradoxically the requirements to manage, within an agenda such as this, are increased rather than diminished. Fundamentally, we must question where do the leadership capacity and capabilities come from to serve and drive forward this agenda?

The United Kingdom's National Health Service (NHS) represents an interesting and valuable perspective on the application of NPM philosophies within a large and complex organisational setting. Within what is often cited as Europe's single largest employer, there has been, as was discussed in our previous chapter, considerable reform agenda in place over a period of some two decades, under the aegis of two separate political administrations. In 2002 the importance of leadership within the ongoing reform aspirations was highlighted by the creation of the NHS Leadership Centre. Although clearly still an organisation in evolution, the centre has articulated a mission that sees three priority areas for leadership development being identified: these being Personal Qualities, Setting Direction and Delivering the Service (NHS Modernisation Agency 2003).

An interesting perspective on this articulation of intent is provided by independently sourced research focusing upon leadership capacity within the NHS, using as benchmark data, perspectives gained from the wider UK public service environment. The researchers argue that 'leadership effectiveness is ultimately determined by the perceptions of staff' and that in an organisation as large and complex as the NHS, perceptions are critical to actually establishing credibility for moving forward the considerable reform agenda that the Blair government has set in train (Alimo-Metcalfe 2003: 29). The areas of greatest concern identified through this work, suggested that within the NHS there was a perception that those who were seen to be leaders were least effective at:

- 'inspiring others;
- supporting a developmental culture;
- showing genuine concern;
- encouraging change;
- being honest and consistent;
- acting with integrity.'

(Alimo-Metcalfe 2003: 29)

Perhaps the most striking message which can be usefully extracted from this listing is that those who are seen as leaders do not appear to be perceived as being closely engaged with the key change agenda that NHS reform, and its NPM underpinnings, regard as crucial. Leaders, who are not seen as supporting a cultural shift or being receptive to change, suggest that the traits and behaviours adopted by them have rather more alignment with the perspective of the service manager.

Here we have the single most important issue of definition, for when we refer to public service leaders, or even engage in research upon their behaviours and traits, what is typically found is a pre-dominance of managerialist attitudes and behaviours, which do not reflect the pre-eminence of a change or transformational agenda. The dilemma within NPM, is that when the spotlight is turned upon the capacity of public service organisations to transform themselves (the creation of the NHS Leadership Centre being an ongoing example of transformation having an explicit linkage to the leadership agenda), too often the reflection is dissonant, change is not enacted with conviction or credibility and the NPM proposition is, itself, undermined. The message we must take from this is clear: added to the seven key doctrines of NPM must surely be a requirement that appropriate leadership is in place, at key milestone phases, to ensure that change is enacted.

How then might the 'eighth doctrine' of NPM be articulated and contextualised for a diverse sector that has grown accustomed to, although not necessarily comfortable with, ongoing change? Reflecting on the starting-point for this chapter, where Kotter set out his view that leadership was not something to be regarded as mysterious or heroic, what does it actually mean to lead public services through a period of change and consolidation? A valuable perspective on this question is provided by Feiner who picks up and develops Kotter's argument:

'... leadership is not about great strategy, great oratory, great heroism or great charisma. Although leaders devote enormous amounts of time to creating the right strategy for the enterprise – a process that is critical to organisational success – formulating strategies is far easier than implementing them. Leadership is more about managing relationships. Success takes intuitive or learned knowledge of how exactly to lead people – how to execute through them, motivate and empower them.'

(Feiner, E. 2000)

Thus Feiner directs us to consider the human interaction and behaviour modification aspects of leadership – which, if we reflect upon the data emerging from the NHS study referred to earlier in this chapter, would appear to be wise advice.

So, to the six doctrines, we add a seventh which is about *leading adaptation*, acknowledging as we surely must, that public services are almost universally people-rich structures. (In Chapter 1 we discussed a perspective on leadership, which we named an enabler perspective of leadership.) To develop and enact the characteristics and principles of NPM requires not only an articulation of intent, but also that those charged with delivering reformed and refocused services, can lead and motivate those within the organisation to adapt their behaviours and possibly even beliefs. Friedman refers to this approach as typifying 'total leadership' which requires of the leaders that they demonstrate authenticity, integrity and creativity:

'Authenticity arises when leaders behave in ways that are consistent with their core values. Leaders must define and articulate a vision that embraces the diverse values and lifestyles of all employees. Their everyday actions must fit their personal values and the core values of the business. They must delegate to cultivate trust, build on strengths and increase commitment to share goals through genuine dialogue with people about whom they care.'

(Friedman 1998)

To take this single point of authenticity, clearly this is a behavioural trait which must be shared across all the various leadership strata of the organisation. Where we have, as many public sector organisations typically do, many thousands of employees, spread across dispersed geographical sites, the impact of a lone authentic leadership figure can be minimal. Thus, an organisational philosophy which is actually *believed* and *adopted* across the organisation is key, for without it, the critical stamp of authenticity is likely to be elusive.

To turn to Friedman's focus upon integrity as being a key component of an overarching leadership model:

'Integrity arises when different aspects of life fit together coherently and consistently. How do leaders achieve this? They must take responsibility for capturing synergies across all aspects of their lives, at work, at home, in the

community and in themselves . . .. They must set, maintain and respect the
boundaries that enable value to be created at work . . ..'

(Friedman 2002: 10)

Such a viewpoint links closely to the increasingly high-profile agenda
of 'work life balance' and just as importantly in this context, to the
ability of leaders to be personally adaptive. The demands of senior-
level leadership roles in public services have escalated considerably
under the influence of NPM and the attrition rates are arguably in
alignment with those of the commercial sector. This is complicated
still further by the limitations to personal integrity that can arise out of
the NPM adherence to external performance monitoring of service
performance.

The third 'ingredient' of a NPM recipe for 'total leadership' is that
of demonstrating and encouraging creativity that Friedman argues
arises when:

'. . . leaders question traditional assumptions and experiment with how things
are done, embracing and initiating change. They need to rethink that means
by which work gets done in ways that force better results. They should
experiment with new work methods and communication tools.'

(Friedman 2002: 10)

Clearly this links closely to the adaptive leadership agenda which has
been posited in this chapter. Critically for leadership within a NPM
context to be effective it must demonstrate a willingness to embrace a
creative agenda and encourage others to do so also. This final part of
the 'puzzle', it can be argued, represents the difference between NPM
as a reform agenda, and NPM as a transformational and delivery-
focused activity. A passion for informed creativity and the skills to
communicate this to, and enthuse others with, a similar commitment
is arguably the single greatest challenge for senior-level public service
leaders today.

NPM IN ACTION – BRISBANE CITY COUNCIL

Australia, together with its near neighbour New Zealand, has had a
considerable influence upon the emergence of the NPM perspective
on the management of public services. As a country the geographical
spread is immense, yet much of the population is centred around
urban areas mainly located on the eastern seaboard. Its model of
governance is undoubtedly complex with Commonwealth (central),
State (sub-central) and local authorities all having a share in the service
delivery model. Analysis of the Australian experience provides
valuable insight into the opportunities for service reform that stems
from a NPM approach whilst all the while highlighting the pivotal role
that leadership plays in actually achieving delivery of change agenda.

Possibly one of the most interesting examples to emerge has been that of Brisbane City Council, an authority serving almost one million residents which has responsibility for services as diverse as public health, public transport, water and sewage and bushland preservation. In the mid-1990s the authority articulated an ambitious reform agenda which was based upon the key principles of NPM, that services should have citizen focus designed into them and that performance and satisfaction levels should rise whilst cost allied to service transaction should fall. This reformist agenda was developed and communicated by the Chief Executive Officer, Robert Carter, and championed vigorously by the elected officers of the council, in particular the elected mayor, Jim Sorley. So from the outset there was clearly close alignment between the strategic and operational aspects of the council and the political dimension to whom they were accountable. Allied to this, Carter recruited to key leadership roles people whom he assessed as exemplifying the 'total leadership' skill set that was discussed previously in this chapter. Together they analysed the scope and scale of the challenges facing the council:

'In 1995, the Council addressed the issue that customers found the organisation difficult to do business with, due to the complex organisational structure and a tendency for work units to operate as independent silos. An integrated customer service project was formed to draw together service delivery across the organisation, focusing initially on counter and telephone services. Council had, at that time, 620 phone numbers listed in the "White Pages" and provided counter service through seven customer service centres. The project recommended a concept of seamless, anywhere, anytime service delivery through one-stop shop counter and telephone services and a variety of self-help facilities.

It was envisaged that the customer would be able to contact the council via a range of channels including the telephone, mail and internet from locations including home, libraries and community centres and could access the full range of council services without having to know or understand the organisational structure. This would be achieved through integrated service delivery processes and systems that would provide a consistent window into the council.'

(Milner 2002: 65)

The project that was articulated in 1995 represented a profound challenge to the way that the council and those employed within it had been accustomed to working and represents, to a very great extent, the global challenge of attempting to lead in a NPM environment. What Carter and his colleagues aspired to do, was not only to change the structures of the council but, fundamentally, also they sought to transform the experience of doing business with Brisbane-delivered public services.

The vision set out by Carter and Sorley was fused into a set of service transformation projects, each with an identified leader.

Remembering that the adoption and implementation phase for this project was the 1990s, the decision to move to a corporate call centre approach, was, at this point in time, demonstrating high levels of creativity in public service terms. The central planks of service redesign were supported by Carter's repeatedly articulated view that successful implementation was entirely dependent upon having the right people in place and the right processes and systems to support them. With hindsight it is possible to view how absolutely key those recruited into leadership roles proved to be in delivering successful implementation and continuing development of what became known as the 'integrated customer service project'.

To consider what was being undertaken, the decision to move to a call centre required that detailed consideration needed to be given to the ways in which over 2,000 separate service offerings could be made to the public:

> 'Every telephone number and customer process incorporated into the call centre was subject to business process re-engineering analysis. The problems experienced by customers were reflected in the multiple iterations experienced during redesign. Many areas considered that their enquiries were too complex to be handled from the call centre and a number of operational areas subsequently struggled to identify irrefutable answers to the information required . . . such as:
>
> ■ What questions do customers ask?
> ■ What are the correct answers?
> ■ Where was this information held?
> ■ Why are customers given different answers on different days and by different people?
> ■ What is the totality of the information the customer needs to know?'
>
> (Milner 2002: 67)

Such a set of questions could and probably should underpin any citizen-facing reform agenda. The particular value of considering Brisbane City Council within a NPM allied leadership context, is that it represents an example of creative practice which can benefit from longitudinal analysis. The culture built by Carter, of citizen-focused emphasis upon continuous review of service, has been successful, the call centre application discussed above has matured and added considerable internet-based access to its portfolio. Key leaders involved in the original championing of profound change have moved on, but then so too has the organisation. Within NPM terms, Brisbane has developed the leadership capacity to exemplify a public service organisation which is both reflective and adaptive. The initial challenges presented by Carter and colleagues were radical, but couched in terms which respected a service ethos and the values of key employee groups. The articulation of the vision into a series of projects was also, in retrospect, highly significant. Whilst Carter was the strategic and operational lead for all activities within the council, his project-oriented approach allowed others to develop and provide key leadership skills which built across the organisation, strengthening its capacity to develop and demonstrate adaptive and creative traits at all levels.

Brisbane City Council offers us key opportunities to learn from the positive alignment of a change agenda and appropriate leadership at all levels of the organisation. What we can also take from it, with some degree of certainty, is that here is a NPM case study that represents significant 'return on investment' in terms of service transformation and the delivery of change. The role of leadership within this process is possible to plot over time, from the original articulation of the vision for change, made by both the political and the executive leaders of the council, through to the working through of a variety of change projects that linked into the overall plan. Critically, throughout a process which was far from pain-free, where there was considerable dislocation of staff groups from established roles, the authenticity and credibility of those in leadership roles rarely appeared to be challenged. Critical to attaining such a position of relative strength, is that the leadership team within Brisbane was coalesced around a shared vision of what the council should be and that there was little evidence of dilution or of undermining of this view. Success within Brisbane stemmed certainly from focusing upon people and processes and leading in ways which made organisational change relevant to those employed within the organisation and those who accessed and used services.

ADAPTIVE LEADERSHIP

Our consideration of the juxtapositioning of leadership and the NPM dynamic led to a view being expressed that what public services actually required was leaders who were, above all, *adaptive*. By this what was meant was that they were capable of developing, communicating and delivering organisational change with a high degree of emphasis being placed upon ensuring that all stakeholders within such processes felt involved and possibly even empowered. To set this within a wider context for public services, such an approach represents a completely different direction to the diverse routes of Machiavellian-style leadership and Weber-influenced bureaucracy. Understanding the mind-sets most commonly associated with the two most widely known 'leadership styles' represents an important point of reference when seeking to understand the challenges of trying to lead in an adaptive and enabling way.

To Machiavelli we must defer, as Crainer argues, as the champion of leadership through cunning and intrigue, indeed Machiavellian leadership philosophy is underpinned by a belief that force will always triumph over reason (Crainer 1996: 10). Extreme as such a perspective may appear, it is possible, even in the 21st century, to observe organisations where leadership is delivered via dictat; where bullying may be the norm rather than an aberration; and where internal politics dominate to such an extent that the achievement of external focus is seriously compromised. Those who have given close scrutiny to the works of Machiavelli can argue with some degree of certainty that such an approach, whilst often blunt and possibly even brutal, has been demonstrably successful within certain contexts. However, such an approach, whilst being both ethically and morally questionable, is also unlikely to deliver organisational success in the longer term. For, with such an emphasis upon intrigue and the establishment and defence of power bases, there is actually little capacity available for continuing to scan externally to ensure that a range of potential 'futures' is kept continuously under review. Of course, allied to this, there should also be a widely shared understanding and sense of responsibility for the need for an organisation to continually review the way it is organised to 'do business'.

Understandably, Machiavellian approaches to leadership, whilst certainly reflecting some of the more questionable human traits and behaviours, have fallen from favour in the last three decades. However, it would be naïve in the extreme to suggest that simply because they are not held up for plaudits, they do not exist.

Sitting at the other extreme of leadership theory but, paradoxically perhaps, having in common with Machiavellian approaches the predilection for establishing control, are the theories of bureaucracy, most famously espoused by Max Weber. For public service organisations, the Weberian model of organisational structure and operation was one that had grown and prospered over decades, if not centuries. The emphasis within Weberian theory being not upon leadership, nor indeed management, but crucially instead being the concept of *administration*.

The public service reforms of the 1980s and the development of NPM subsequent to these represent an ongoing effort to dismantle bureaucratic structures and traditions, and with them potentially the attitudes and behaviours of those employed within public services. Fundamental to understanding the challenges represented here we must address exactly what it is that typically characterises bureaucratic organisations. In this respect Loffler and Klages's summary is helpful, in as much as they suggest that NPM represents a challenge to classical hierarchical structures and to traditional principles of public service employment such as lifelong employment and salary related to tenure rather than performance (Loffler and Klages 1995). Developing a leadership style that can challenge and move forward such a strong cultural setting represents one of the defining challenges of public service leadership today. That this is a defensible view, over two decades on from the first articulation of NPM, when one might reasonably have expected that the structural and cultural changes required had already been achieved, is an indication of the challenges of becoming an effective and adaptive leader in much of the public service environment.

Consideration of the Machiavellian and Weberian perspectives reminds us once again that the scope and scale of enacting wide-ranging public service reform through the deployment of effective leadership is, at the very least, a difficult task. Having set out a perspective that possibly the single most important trait within a NPM reform agenda, is that adaptive leadership should be present, there is a need to focus upon what this actually means. When referring to adaptive behaviours and characteristics, what do we actually mean? One of the most influential commentators on the area of leadership, Warren Bennis, provides valuable insight and perspective on the roles that effective leaders must adopt and the personal characteristics and traits they must exemplify. Whilst of course, Bennis's 'recipe' approach may lack some of the subtle nuances that the public service environment might well require, it does give us a sense of what adaptive leadership should actually look like in practice:

'The first ingredient of leadership is *guiding vision*. The leader has a clear idea of what he wants to do – professionally and personally – and the strength to persist in the face of setbacks, even failures. Unless you know where you are going, and why, you cannot possibly get there.

The second basic ingredient of leadership is *passion* – the underlying passion for the promises of life, combined with a very particular passion for a vocation, a profession, and a course of action. The leader loves what he is doing and loves doing it. Tolstoy said that hopes are the dreams of the waking man. Without hope, we cannot survive, much less progress. The leader who communicates passionately gives hope and inspiration to other people.

The next basic ingredient of leadership is *integrity*. I think there are three essential parts of integrity: self-knowledge, candour and maturity.

"Know thyself" was the inscription over the Oracle at Delphi. And it is still the most difficult task any of us faces. But until you truly know yourself, strengths and weaknesses, know what you want to do and why you want to do it, you cannot succeed in any but the most superficial sense of the word . . .

Candour is the key to self-knowledge. Candour is based in honesty of thought and action, a steadfast devotion to principle and fundamental soundness and wholeness . . .

Maturity is important to a leader because leading is not simply showing the way or issuing orders. Every leader needs to have experienced and grown through following – learning to be dedicated, observant, capable of working with and learning from others . . .. Having located these in himself, he can encourage them in others.

Integrity is the basis of *trust*, which is not as much an ingredient of leadership as it is a product. It is one quality that cannot be acquired, but must be earned. It is given by co-workers and followers, and without it the leader can't function.

Two more basic ingredients of leadership are *curiosity* and *daring*. The leader wonders about everything, wants to learn as much as he can, is willing to take risks, experiment, try new things. He does not worry about failure but embraces errors, knowing he will learn from them.'

(Bennis 1998: 41–2)

The amalgam of personal traits and public demonstration that Bennis argues for does represent a synthesis of the qualities of the adaptive leader. Critically too it represents a further stage in the differentiation between what it may mean to be a manager, or even a bureaucrat in modern public services. The crucial areas of difference, which Bennis articulates, it must be noted, primarily for a commercial sector audience, are similarly helpful in gauging not only the characteristics and personality traits of a leader, but also, what the leader actually *does:*

- The manager administers; the leader innovates;
- The manager is a copy; the leader is an original;
- The manager maintains; the leader develops;
- The manager focuses on systems and structure; the leader focuses on people;
- The manager relies on control; the leader inspires trust;
- The manager has a short-range view; the leader has a long-range perspective;
- The manager asks how and when; the leader asks what and why;
- The manager always has his eye on the bottom line, the leader has his eye on the horizon;
- The manager imitates, the leader originates;
- The manager accepts the status quo; the leader challenges it;
- The manager is the classic good soldier, the leader is his own person.'

(Bennis 1998: 44–5)

The adaptive traits highlighted here have considerable resonance with aspects of the development agenda discussed earlier in this chapter, set out by the NHS Leadership Centre. Fundamentally what we see is further evidence that leading and managing whilst potentially within the remit of a single individual require complex and different skill sets and behaviours. In subsequent chapters our focus will be upon testing out, within largely applied contexts, the extent to which an adaptive approach is always possible within the political and policy frameworks which govern so much of our public service environments.

CHANGING RULES AND ROUTINES – THE LEADERSHIP CHALLENGE

Having navigated our way through the emergence of NPM as an underpinning driver for public service change and highlighted the adaptive leadership concept as being pivotal in developing a leadership paradigm for this context, it is important to turn our attention to the notion of change itself. Change and change management are so often discussed within modern organisations, that it is possible to form a view that the only thing that one can be absolutely sure of, is that change or a perception of the need for change are always going to be on the public service agenda. In part it is possible to argue that the passion for change stems, in large part, from a perception held by politicians, that public service organisations remain locked into a Weberian bureaucratic model of practice.

Such a perception, even some 25 years on from the wide-ranging reforms pioneered by the administrations of Thatcher and Reagan, is indicative of an underpinning current of opinion that holds that public services remain essentially inefficient and resource-wasteful. It must also be noted that public services find themselves all too often in the spotlight simply because they represent one of the softer 'targets' for politicians to enter into debate over. So for public services globally, the pressure to engage with change is ever present. As was discussed in the case of Brisbane City Council, the change processes have represented a shared vision owned by politicians and executive leaders.

Careful analysis of the public service operating environment suggests that there are typically two major change agendas that are associated with change and modernisation. The first can usefully be termed as *rules*; changing rules relates fundamentally to consideration of both the formal and informal *rules of engagement* which govern the extent to which public service organisations can be encouraged or required to work differently. Challenging established rules typically involves looking at the way in which services are designed and delivered and questioning whether existing structures or even barriers remain appropriate. Rules of course, particularly in the area of revenue and benefits, may also bring into play the reality that the rules being discussed actually exist in legislation. Leaders who challenge rules such as these will typically require high-level political sign-up if progress is to be made and change actively pursued. More typically perhaps, a policy framework may emerge which then gives service leaders the opportunity to embrace a change agenda that has already been articulated.

A major challenge to public service rules is discussed in Chaper 3, around the example in Australia of the Centrelink organisation, which represented the creation of a single point of contact for a range of benefits and educational services. Picking up on a theme emerging in this chapter of Australia being in the vanguard of NPM reform, we should also consider the opening up of its revenue services to incorporate aspects of activity relating to work and pensions. Such an unpacking of previously apparently indissoluble barriers has inspired the United Kingdom's Treasury Department, in 2003, to set in train a review which has its underpinning hypothesis that more cost-effective and citizen-friendly services might emerge from following the Australian model. To date, it is too early to posit a view as to how such a change is being responded to at a leadership level within the organisations affected by the review. However, a helpful perspective on this rule-change challenge for leadership is provided by Nicholson-O'Brien in reviewing the attitudes to change adopted by the government of Canada, who argues that the only approach possible has been to champion the 'planned abandonment of whatever no longer serves us well' (Milner 2002: 89).

A further key strand of this argument around challenges to rules is provided by the acceleration of the involvement of non-governmental providers in the delivery of public services. From the first forays into contracting out of services such as refuse in the early 1980s, we now find, particularly in the USA, that there have been significant moves towards bringing the private and not-for-profit sectors into the service delivery dynamic. The key 'rule' that has been breached here is that which might have held that there remain some services, such as education and social care, that are of such a special nature that they can and should only ever be led, managed and delivered by public service organisations. That there is now widespread adoption of policies, which are designed to facilitate the removal of the delivery aspect from the umbrella of the public service, throws up yet another issue of adaptation for the leadership role working within these contexts.

Fundamentally, what we see in developments such as these can possibly be termed as the rolling out of NPM stage two. By this what is meant is that whilst Hood (1991) and Osborne and Gaebler (1992) set out a vision of NPM which saw public services being designed in different ways and interacting with the citizen in a more focused manner, their paradigm remained principally one which did not challenge the existence of public services as the principal channel of delivery in their own right. However, as practice has evolved and political agendas have developed and matured around this concept of challenging rules, so too there has been something of a paradigm shift, to a position where from a 21st century perspective, what we can actually map, are views emerging which demonstrate close alignment with those of the mid-19th century. NPM stage two suggests, it can reasonably be argued, that public services should only ever be delivered by public bodies where there is demonstrably no other organisation which can do it for the same or lower cost. The concept of government being the facilitator of services, with the majority of provision being located in the charitable or private sectors, is a model which we can see being deployed across the globe, and which, historically speaking, represented the position broadly adopted by the Victorians (Owen 1965).

Setting aside the historical footnote, which whilst interesting in itself, represents a position at a point in time where citizen expectations of public services had no benchmark position to measure against. Where public services find themselves today, is in an environment where in many instances new rules of engagement are evolving all the time. Providing leadership within this scenario requires that the adaptive characteristics discussed previously in this chapter become ever more essential. As the rules have changed, so too have relationships and structures, the routines which have typified public service working have, in many cases, disappeared, as new service models have emerged.

When considering the impact upon leaders and their capacity to lead within this change context, one must understand that leadership roles have possibly never been more key than they are in the shift towards new structural and indeed mental models of working. For those who have held public service roles over considerable periods of time, they may find themselves seeking to lead in situations where both reporting lines and accountability structures have been blurred or even obliterated. Routines, which provide the underpinnings of any service offering, when transferred to a third party provider, are inevitably going to be challenged and/or redesigned. If the service leadership role transfers to the new provider's environment, it is reasonable to anticipate that there can be considerable capacity for disconnection between the leadership style and expectations of the public service environment and those of a contracted provider. Similarly, one can also anticipate that where organisations are gaining public service contracts for service delivery, they may not always have available to them leaders who can demonstrate empathy with the environment in which they are working.

The third element of this leadership theme is that which relates to the leader at one remove. By this what is meant, is that whilst service offerings may be subject to delivery by third parties under managed contracts, those charged with leading the 'facilitating' structures may once again find themselves facing leadership challenges in unfamiliar territory. A little-discussed aspect of leadership development in public services is that of responding to the challenges of delegated delivery and the allied skill sets that may be required. For whilst those occupying operational level leadership roles may have to address issues of dealing with new environments and cultures, the strategic leader is placed in a position of having considerable responsibility and accountability, without necessarily having access to the levers and counter-balances which can bring the capacity for remedial adjustment. Being a public service leader within this scenario is something which is unfamiliar and which does require from those occupying such roles that they have both the confidence and resilience to lead relationships rather than services *per se.*

Possibly one of the best examples of an administration realising that leadership roles in an environment where rules and routines are regularly being tested, is provided by the Canadian government's creation of what it terms the 'Leadership Network'. As discussed by Nicholson-O'Brien, the network which is itself led by one of the country's most senior civil servants, Mary Gusella, is:

'. . . applying a new vision with regard to networks of leaders at all levels for Canada's public service. The Leadership Network (TLN) is about investment by the corporate system in experimenting in new ways to deliver key services.

She (Gusella) notes that public service managers are not accustomed to declaring experimentation as an alternative vision to doing the old things in the old ways. She further rejects the traditional system that rewards technocrats and old-style crisis managers. Her definition of new-style crisis management means having leaders whose decisions deposit us gently ahead of issues.

Gusella and her team are developing a leadership laboratory that invites leaders to create conceptual frameworks to meet their business and leadership challenges. The Leadership Network represents a "safe haven" where leaders can begin to see an ethic of care in action, where mentoring occurs and is prioritised as a developmental activity. Simply put, the philosophy is that if we care for a leader, then they will learn to care for others . . .. She begins with the premise that leaders not only want to do the best that they can do, but that they will raise the bar behaviourally and ethically, when given the right support and opportunity to do so.'

(Milner 2002: 99–100)

An approach such as this represents the first movement towards New Public Leadership emerging as a real agenda item for administrations. Setting aside the fact that for many years there have been well-defined management development programmes, the emphasis here, on leadership and leading in new contexts, represents a key acknowledgement of the fact that the public service leadership challenge has moved centre stage. Critically what it must seek to do, is to engender the adaptive and change orientation traits and behaviours discussed previously within this chapter, in the context of the established rules and routines of public service being set aside as NPM moves into its second phase. Critically, as Milner argues, leadership within these new models of service design and delivery requires a capacity to understand and address the key threats to service quality and improvement agenda that reside in the new structures:

'Governments who advocate the adoption of a position where they are an enabler rather than necessarily a direct provider of public services have typically not acknowledged the fact that they may be absenting themselves from an environment which is most likely to inform their service planning . . . the emphasis to date has been upon ensuring that performance criteria have been put in place, against which even crude measures of baseline performance can be assessed . . .. The challenge and perhaps the critical paradox now is that in a climate when public services are being called upon to innovate and develop new modes of user-centred working, they are increasingly seeing their key employee assets being transferred to agencies or organisations at some remove from their direct control.'

(Milner 2002: 14)

For a leader to operate effectively within this complex environment is surely the largest single leadership challenge that is faced within the public service context. Changing rules and routines whilst apparently straightforward concepts, are in themselves the foundations of all organisational change programmes and map closely against the aspiration to develop new behaviours and cultures. Public service leaders across the world are today seeking to find ways of making new service paradigms work and ensuring that the public service capacity to develop and innovate is not lost in the rush to engage in relationship working with a host of providers for whom innovation, and risks associated with it, are not willingly owned. Whether the implications of removing rules and structural divides are fully considered at a policy level in terms of the type and levels of leadership required to ensure efficacy in the new service environment, is something for which there is little evidence to support a view in the affirmative.

LEADING ORGANISATIONAL CHANGE AND RENEWAL

The final strand in our analysis of the theoretical and applied strands that make critical input to the development of a New Public Leadership paradigm, is that of organisational *renewal*. Stripping away the political rhetoric which often dominates the public service reform domain it is clear that where, for example, the demand for *modernisation* is often the headline, what are actually desired are sustainable and user-centred change practices. It is here that the concept of organisational renewal becomes particularly apposite: for it is in the study of renewal as a consequence of change that occurs over time, that we can see the potential for the achievement of new models of public service.

Perhaps the best advocates for renewal as being a key organisational aspiration are Tushman and O'Reilly who, whilst not overtly addressing a public service audience, do identify key themes which have considerable resonance for this sector (Tushman and O'Reilly 2002). Key to the concept of renewal and its inextricable link to leadership is a recognition that so many change management activities, regardless of the type of organisation within which they are deployed, do not deliver significant benefits over the medium term at the very least. Renewal on the other hand presents change and change practices as being part of a phased continuum, reliant for their articulation and implementation upon effective leadership over the longer term, and which form part of organisational capacity building, in essence equipping organisations with the culture and allied behaviours to address a range of possible futures. Tushman and O'Reilly review the lessons that can be learned from the past and the implications that such analysis can have for those interested in exploring the concept of renewal:

'In the 1980s the business press was filled with accounts of the managerial prowess of firms like Toyota, Apple and People Express. Today People Express is gone, Apple is a shadow of its former self, and European automakers like Mercedes are using Ford, not Toyota, as their benchmark. In the

1980s, managers raced to implement techniques like quality circles, just-in-time inventory, and lean manufacturing. Today we read articles about the failure of Total Quality Management (TQM) and the dangers of reengineered, anorexic organizations . . .

This pattern – success followed by failure; innovation followed by inertia – is common across firms and industries over time. It isn't an American, European or Asian phenomenon; it is a global disease and can strike managers at all levels of organizations . . .

Yet success need not be paralyzing. The most successful firms are able to capture the benefits of short-term advantage even as they build organizational capabilities for long-term strategic renewal. They transform themselves through proactive innovation and strategic change. Proactive firms are able to move from today's strength to tomorrow's strength by setting the pace of innovation in their industries.

To succeed both today and tomorrow, managers must play two different games simultaneously. Firstly they must continually get better at competing in the short-term, which requires increasing the alignment among strategy, people, culture and processes. The efficiency game requires mastering the basics. Yet efficiency alone will not ensure long-term success. In fact today's success may actually increase the chances of tomorrow's failure. For sustainable success, managers must also master another game: understanding how and when to initiate revolutionary innovation and, in turn, revolutionary organizational change.

Organizational renewal demands mastering the dynamics of innovation and organizational change. Great managers are able to manage for today and for tomorrow simultaneously. The ability to play both games is crucial for long-term survival and success. The tools necessary to master these are understandable and implementable by managers everywhere. These tools help managers become architects of their organizations, constantly managing the contexts in which people operate.'

(Tushman and O'Reilly 2002: 2–3)

Whilst acknowledging that much of Tushman and O'Reilly's focus is understandably upon the commercial sector environment, the importance and relevance of what they say to the public service community should not be underestimated. Crucially, the position they articulate shares substantial common ground with public service scenarios internationally. Public services have, only in rare instances such as arguably the Australian example of Centrelink which was discussed earlier in the book, followed a change agenda which promotes addressing the here and now, as well as a range of potential future scenarios simultaneously. Innovation, although typically advocated and lauded, has also tended to be of the short-termist, short-sighted type to which these commentators allude. The role of the manager or leader is, within the renewal context, a critical one, for it is, it would appear, only through sustained leadership input, that the potential for the creation of a culture that is capable of sustaining ongoing innovation can be created.

Adaptive leadership, the theoretical amalgam suggested within this text, would appear to lend itself well to the pursuit of a renewal agenda. What can be usefully drawn from the work of Tushman and O'Reilly as a particular addition to adaptive theme, is their articulation of what it means to be a leader within a renewal context and specific actions that leaders can take to support the promotion of the concept. Critically, they argue, organisational renewal requires what they refer to as 'visionary leaders', a term which requires some further clarification and contextualisation:

> 'Visionary leaders are able to mobilize and sustain energy and activity within an organization by taking specific personal actions. Visionary leaders are not the popular versions of the great speech makers or television personalities. Visionary leadership is not equivalent to charisma. Rather, visionary leaders are able to engage their organization at whatever level they operate . . . they influence their colleagues' values, goals, needs and aspirations through their relentless attention to shaping interpretations and creating a sense of purpose.
>
> Visionary leaders energize the organization and find ways to motivate its members to achieve its goals. They demonstrate empathy, listen, understand and share the feelings of others in the organization. They express their confidence in their own ability and in the ability of others to succeed. They create events to signal and celebrate transitions and turning points, expressing support for individuals grappling with the pressures of stressful change efforts and reinforcing the new vision and culture.
>
> The behaviors associated with visionary leadership support innovation and change in several ways. Visionary leaders provide a psychological focal point for the energies, hopes, and aspirations of people in the organization. They serve as powerful role models whose actions and personal energy demonstrate the desired behaviors. Their behavior is a standard to which others can aspire. Through their commitment, effectiveness and consistency, visionary leaders build a personal bond between themselves and the organization.'
>
> (Tushman and O'Reilly 2002: 186–7)

This undoubtedly challenging view of what it means to be a *leader* amplifies the position outlined by Kotter at the beginning of this chapter which sets the role of a leader apart and different from that of a manager. The development of this position by Tushman and O'Reilly is particularly appropriate in the context of this work more generally, for rather than stating as many commentators on leadership do, that it is critical to acknowledge the role of leaders at all levels of an organisation, they forcibly argue that if the most senior leaders are not working effectively and cohesively to promote and support change and innovation, then there is little that others can achieve. It is possible to argue that it has been the frequent failure to acknowledge the pivotal role played by the most senior leaders that has made public services appear to be laggards in change and innovation processes. It is for this reason that much of this text will concentrate upon leadership as deployed at the most senior levels of public service organisations, for quite simply the authors' critical analysis suggests that is in this area that the opportunities for real development and indeed renewal capacity must be initially nurtured.

Adaptive leadership as articulated within this chapter should therefore be seen as providing the theoretical point of reference for an emergent model of public service activity. Within the context of analysing aspects of practice and of consideration of discrete case studies, the questions we must always return to are those of leadership capacity. Where is it? Is it truly adaptive? Can the leadership styles sustain the management of change and the development of a culture that is capable of embracing innovative practices over time? As we have seen, there is no single or simple theoretical model which can be mapped across to the public sector setting; then possibly the best articulation we can arrive at is, that if New Public Management can be said to be an organic and evolving concept, then allied to it must be an emergent New Public Leadership model. It is the intention of subsequent chapters to provide both context and opportunities for learning that will enable a reflective stance to be taken on this view of leaders and leadership within public services. With this goal in mind, it is useful to consider the perspective provided by Heifetz and Laurie:

> 'Leadership . . . requires a learning strategy. A leader from above or below with or without authority has to engage people in confronting the challenge, adjusting their values, changing perspectives, and learning new habits. To an authoritative person who prides himself on his ability to tackle hard problems, this shift may come as a rude awakening. But it should also ease the burden of having to know all the answers and bear all the load . . .. The adaptive demands of our time require leaders who take responsibility without waiting for revelation or request.'
>
> (Heifetz and Laurie 1997: 197)

Within this context of adaptive and innovation-focused leadership, it is helpful to consider the views of one of the most influential public service practitioners currently operating in this arena. Dawn Nicholson-O'Brien, a senior figure in the civil service of Canada, has been charged with developing innovation and allied leadership strategies which will best serve the needs of her ambitious and diverse nation. Her 'voice on leadership', a contribution developed specifically for this text, is an important one for any audience interested in understanding the challenges and possibilities associated with what we have termed adaptive, new public leadership.

LEADERSHIP: ESTABLISHING DREAMS WITH DEADLINES 'COMMENTS BY DAWN NICHOLSON-O'BRIEN'

Today, wherever citizens around the globe reside, we are the beneficiaries of personal, collective and institutional leadership exercised in innumerable spheres. In Canada, our society is reaping the dividends of a high quality of life and of a knowledge-based society forged in the post-WWII era. It is not sufficient, however, to live off of this 'accrued interest'. Looking to the future of Canadian society and to the future of the world community, investments are being undertaken to create new realities in human experience.

Many new discoveries are forcing us to rethink our beliefs about the universe and our place in it. Leadership, therefore, is rooted in creating the future, informed by a guiding sense of purpose, initiating norm-altering behaviours, and engaging new culture carriers across domestic and global networks as we do so. This entails ensuring that favourable mutations or new ideas are carried forward as a living legacy through small world networks.

Leaders and innovators lower barriers of all kinds to permit a higher rate of disruptive innovation, thereby actively disturbing the present in the service of the future.

THE FUTURE IS CREATED IN THE PRESENT

We might well ask, when does leadership occur? How do we innovate continuously to create the future?

Leadership emerges when we are discussing a 'desired future', one that as yet does not exist. The future exists only as a result of what we initiate today, using the past not as an immutable point of departure. Leaders are history-makers or history-breakers, going beyond boundary innovations to create new worlds. Leaders are learners who behave with integrity. They mobilise the collective intelligence of entire organisations, networks, and societies, thereby creating audacious goals and delivering incredible outcomes. They are serial innovators not just episodic innovators responding to crises of the day. In Canada, one of our national pastimes is the game of hockey. There are two ways to play the game: to sit ringside as an armchair critic and to comment on each play or to play the game 'on the ice'. Leaders, in my experience, are always playing on the ice, taking risks and learning from challenges. They do not simply come up with new ideas or new dreams – they set dreams with deadlines and bring them to fruition.

In November of 2001, in my capacity as the Senior Visiting Fellow, Innovation, at the Canadian Centre for Management Development, I was asked to develop proposals that would help the Public Service of

Canada to innovate. The outcome, announced in February of 2003, was the creation of innovation incubators to produce results for Canadians in a number of priority areas. (See the website at www. innovation.ccmd-ccg.gc.ca for details.) After conducting research into private and public sector practices in some of the most innovative organisations in the world, it was my pleasure to advance an innovation meritocracy where employees across the country, together with citizens, developed 500 proposals to innovate in the public interest. These proposals were judged in May of 2003 by a distinguished panel of Canada's innovators. Strategic investments were made in the winning pilot projects. With the development of the related infrastructure, the Blue Ribbon Panel, the supporting secretariat and the budget, we succeeded in doing what many thought was at best a pipe-dream.

Today, one of the projects is making policy centres in various parts of government aware of the needs of offenders' families so that resources can be devoted, on a strategic basis, to services tailored to their needs. Those involved are united in efforts to ensure that families of offenders do not get pulled into the downward economic, educational and emotional spirals that often result in subsequent generations engaging in a life of crime and in the resultant loss of human potential. The human and economic costs associated with the incarceration of one person and other costs in the justice system – if averted with this incubator – would more than justify the investment made in the entire initiative. And, the resulting partnerships and networks across society provide the communities and families with the means to own their innovative solutions and to assume control over their destinies.

NORM-ALTERING BEHAVIOURS

In governments we are fortunate to work on extraordinary endeavours like the eradication of child poverty, of planetary scourges like cancer and AIDS, and on other issues that matter to people and that directly affect the quality of life. Equally, we must deal with questions on the frontiers of science, technology and international affairs, or the supranational space. There are few countries in the world that do not, for example, have a patent act of some sort to protect intellectual property, designed to deal with things that may be invented in the future. Leaders in all sectors of society are being called upon to decide the future of various ideas whose dimensions are not merely extensions of the known but extend to the great unknown. How we formulate policy today on space exploration, on computer avatars, on stem cell or proteomics research or on medical treatments will determine human well-being into the future.

In nature, microbiologists have shown that both the frequency and density of mutations increase, as evolutionary challenges become more complex. In a governance context, we cannot disembody discoveries from people. Thus, where we have leaders who are actively scanning for new patterns, anomalies and for what I call extremophiles or odd-ball developments outside of the norm, we find leaders who foster constructive destruction and experimentation. They create open-ended processes for human discovery and for norm-altering outcomes and behaviours by encouraging the unthinkable. They create pockets of intellectual freedom and learning as a commitment to the realisation of dreams and innovation that extend beyond our times.

It is the nature of life that improbable things will happen. Leaders in organisations like Canada's National Research Council and the new National Institute for Nanotechnology, or, in Canada's Business Development Bank, have created new scientific business lines, health prospects and entrepreneurial networks that are shaping Canada's future. Fifty years from now, the next generation of citizens will be able to trace specific developments in Canadian and global societies back to these hothouses for innovation. Governments and successful norm-altering leaders and innovators are creating a biological approach to renewal that is supplanting the mechanical and outdated notion of 'machinery of government'. Organisations of human beings, formerly seen as well-oiled machinery, and strategy, seen as a kind of machine tool, are being replaced by 'strategy as biology'. Human beings are to be perceived as they are – as members of human networks and of evolving communities with multiple identities.

NATURE'S PROTÉGÉS

Governments have learned that there is no duly constituted 'depart-ment of good ideas', policy shop or agency that can meet the challenges of the modern world alone. No single leader or organisation can be literate in every domain of knowledge today but leaders can stimulate access to ideas, create networks across societies and very deliberately assemble teams, partnerships and markets for ideas that are diverse. The public good is always being altered and redefined as governments adapt to externalities. Adaptive leaders seek ideas from all parts of society and in the venerable tradition of the Olympics they encourage friendly competition in their own organisations to ensure that citizens receive the best value for their investments. The call to achieve our vital design as human beings and the enhancement of the public good is not the exclusive purview of governments. Thus, col-laborative leadership with people in all parts of society and around the globe often results in seeing what has not been seen before and in making new priorities visible through culture carriers who foster renewal via their respective networks.

Organisations and societies that serve as an innovation search party – where innovation is derived from robust portfolios of disruptive ideas and where the connoisseurs of ideas are paired with the creators of ideas – are nature's protégés. Each country and each government, like any ecosystem, has its own 'habitat specialists' who possess extensive knowledge of their native environment or country. Biology evolves and adapts rapidly to meet new challenges. In biology-inspired networks, operating with high levels of trust and information-sharing, we are seeing solutions created for what were previously regarded as intractable problems. This involves citizen-led campaigns to eliminate the use of landmines or networks like the International Knowledge Management Forum associated with Canada's International Development Research Centre, creating innovative solutions for the developing world. Governments around the globe, for example, in their role as tax collectors, are finding ways to create incentives for good environmental practices intended to meet the requirements of the Kyoto Accord.

Self-organisation and bureaucracy are not binary states any more than mature governments and new innovation incubators are binary states. They are inter-related and interdependent. The biological flexibility or plasticity that comes with human networks carrying new ideas around the globe and incorporating favourable mutations is built on the foundation code of existing laws, policies and practices, in a symphony of renewal.

CHAPTER 6

CASES IN SUCCESSFUL LEADERSHIP

INTRODUCTION

All three of the case studies in this chapter contain an example of successful managerial leadership. The leaders concerned managed to bring about substantial change and radical improvement. Two of the cases show how change was only achieved despite trade union resistance. The cases also show how old welfare state thinking was being challenged and how a new welfare state was emerging. In this sense, the case studies contain evidence of leaders facilitating the adaptation of the welfare state to the new circumstances of the 21st century.

The first case of leadership was essentially about the attempt by a council to avoid a financial crisis and facing union resistance when it moved away from a commitment to no compulsory redundancy. The second case concerns a local authority in London that adopted a new strategic vision of serving its local community and transformed its performance in only 3 years. The third case was a merger of two government services in pursuit of a new concept of providing services to job seekers. Each of the cases highlighted a different leadership challenge. The first required managerial leaders to take responsibility for a problem that had to be solved before the council could proceed with a change programme for becoming innovative and modernised. In the second case the managerial leader was recruited to help the council to articulate a vision and a programme of change. In the last of the three cases the leadership challenge was to 'front' the vision articulated by politicians and loyally to turn that vision into reality. The challenge in each case was different because the circumstances of leadership were different.

In the light of the novelty of the changes being attempted in the public services and the resistance to change that is occurring, leadership is at times risky and demanding for top managers in the public services. We have already noted Heifetz and Linsky's (2002) analysis of adaptive change as being experimental. The managerial leader who experiments and fails can expect to be criticised by politicians and the media for wasting public money and taking chances. The managerial leaders in our cases did not fail, but they needed to be resilient as well as energetic to cope with the personal dimension of leadership.

All of the cases show the managerial leaders achieving change with the support of elected politicians and we think also show the managerial leaders exercising political skills. Public services organisations are powerfully influenced by the fact that government provides and controls the funding of public services. In consequence, what managerial leaders do is inherently political. They have to pay attention to what political leaders want and expect. They also have to help elected politicians turn political vision, based on ideological convictions, into organisational changes. Political leaders require effective managerial leaders for the delivery of policies. There is a state of interdependence between elected politicians and managerial leaders.

Managerial leaders in all public sector organisations have to pay attention to politicians, but they vary a great deal in terms of their level of direct contact with the elected politicians. This has a major influence on the types of working relationship that political and managerial leaders are able to develop with one another.

As in the past, the public elects politicians to represent them and pursue their interests and aspirations. However, in the search for public services that are more responsive to the needs of the public, politicians have been giving managers more responsibility for the performance of their organisations. One consequence of this is that managerial leaders no longer simply, or only, implement the policies of the politicians (did they ever?). They now have more explicit autonomy, but this is combined with increased accountability through performance management systems, and it requires managerial leaders to become more skilled at getting political support for their plans and actions. We would emphasise our conclusion that top managers in the public services must generate the support of the politicians if they are to act as leaders (Heymann 1987; Moore 1995). Moreover, within a democratic system, this situation requires managers to figure out how their plans and actions can be fitted into the political agenda. While this brings about continuity between the priorities of the elected politicians and the plans and actions of managerial leaders, which is essential for a public service in a democracy, it also makes managerial leaders vulnerable to the accusation that they have become 'political'. This, then, defines the contradictory terrain of the 'new political management' in the modern public services.

CASE OF JOHN FOSTER AT MIDDLESBROUGH COUNCIL

John Foster was described as being 'a moderniser before the phrase was invented' (The MJ, 10–16 November 2000). He joined Middlesbrough Council as managing director and then became its Chief Executive. He was there for five years from the beginning of 1998 to the end of 2002, having been headhunted and offered the top management job in the winter of 1997. He left to become the new Chief Executive at Wakefield City Council, in January 2003, a job which was described as 'one of the most challenging in local government' (The MJ, 24 October 2002). The headlines for The MJ read, 'Foster lured to Wakefield by change agenda pledge'. John had been headhunted because of what he had achieved at Middlesbrough Council. 'Mr Foster, 52, told The MJ that at Middlesbrough he had helped "'turn a failing authority into a high performing one" . . .'.

In December 2002 an Audit Commission report on the comprehensive performance assessment scores and analysis of performance for single-tier authorities and county councils in England stated that Middlesbrough was rated a 'good' council. This put the council in the top half of the 150 councils that had been placed in one of the five CPA categories, which ranged from 'poor' to 'excellent'. According to the same report,

> 'Good councils tend to have strong services overall and know where they need to make improvements. These councils provide effective leadership and management. Good councils have high levels of ambition and are mostly focused on what matters to their communities.'
>
> (Audit Commission, Comprehensive Performance Assessment, Local Government National Report, December 2002: 3; downloaded from Audit Commission website http://www.audit-commission.gov.uk)

This might be seen as a public endorsement for John's stewardship of the council's management. Certainly, the Audit Commission's corporate assessment of Middlesbrough Council was very positive, as indicated by this extract:

> 'Middlesbrough Council is highly ambitious . . .. The council has shown boldness and imagination in embracing the modernisation agenda . . .. The key improvements for driving improvement are mostly in place. Key strengths include a strong corporate culture that is becoming increasingly performance-driven, a strategic network of partnerships geared towards delivering agreed priorities, sound financial management, and intelligent use of external procurement arrangements.'
>
> (Middlesbrough Council, December 2002: 4).

The reference to sound financial management is especially interesting in the light of the situation John found at the council in 1998.

Beginning in a crisis

The year 1997 was a significant time nationally. There had been a change of national government, 'and the new Labour Government was beginning to spell out to local government what it expected in terms of modernisation and change'. This meant that as John took up his new post there were the beginnings of the debate around a range of modernisation issues in local government (best value, political management, ethical standards, etc.). This was, according to John, 'an interesting time'.

Middlesbrough Council recruited John Foster because it needed to make changes. Prior to his appointment, the leader of the council commissioned Price Waterhouse Coopers, to do a review of the senior management of the organisation. The review was extremely critical. The council accepted the main recommendations of the report and agreed to appoint a new managing director. PWC were retained to undertake the search and selection for the post and John was subsequently appointed.

> 'I arrived at the beginning of 1998 knowing that I had been brought in as a "change agent" to use the jargon. I knew that they wanted me to restructure their top management arrangements, and I was okay about that.'

While he was aware of the changes the council wanted in management arrangements, he was, at the time he accepted the job, unaware of the details of a pending financial crisis. That he did become aware of the financial crisis, and aware very early after he had accepted the job, reflects less on his qualities as a visionary leader than on his painstaking analysis and evaluation of documents prior to taking up his new position in February 1998.

> 'I asked the then Director of Finance during the Christmas period to let me have some copies of his detailed budget assumptions and supporting papers. I asked for these things before I started so I had the opportunity of the Christmas period of '97 to understand the detail. I spent December going through all of his papers, at the end of which, in January, I contacted the Director of Finance and said I wasn't happy about the financial implications I was gleaning from the various reports, I would need to have a meeting with him before I arrived, which I did and arranged. At the meeting he began to spell out what I had deduced from my analysis of his reports, that basically the Council had no money, and that they were spending well beyond their means. They had taken no serious steps to deal with the problem, even though there were District Audit management statements going back to the previous year that indicated warning signals that the budget was out of control, and that the Council needed to take steps to remedy it.'

He concluded that, to all intents and purposes, the council was bankrupt. How had it happened? Discussing the situation just after leaving Middlesbrough Council, John referred to two explanations offered by other local authority Chief Executives of the events when Cleveland

County Council was abolished in 1996 and replaced by new unitary authorities. The first was that only Middlesbrough of the four new unitary authorities was committed to avoiding redundancy of Cleveland County Council employees at all costs. The other new unitary authorities made their recruitment and workforce decisions knowing that Middlesbrough would absorb all the employees that were surplus to their requirements. John's view was that the Middlesbrough Chief Executive and chief officers ended up with heavy costs in their management structures as a result of their handling of the situation at the time.

Essentially, we can see the abolition of the county council as creating an issue that was formed by a tension between Middlesbrough Council's commitment to a traditional value of no compulsory redundancies, and a desire to provide modern public services that involves putting the citizens as taxpayers and consumers first. The traditional value meant being ready to take on all surplus employees, whereas the modern value meant having regard to service requirements when making HR decisions.

The commitment to no compulsory redundancy seems to have combined with and reinforced a problem of structural conservatism. Cleveland County Council was based in Middlesbrough. Although it was being abolished, Middlesbrough still wanted to be the dominant town in the political world of Teesside. So:

> 'When Cleveland County Council dissolved, there was a view I think, which was both a political view and a senior managers' view, that Middlesbrough would take on the mantle of the "big town" in Governance terms. And what that meant in practice was that, at a time when the other new unitary authorities were spending time preparing for their new status in terms of what their budgets were likely to be, what their organisational shape should be, what their resources were likely to be, Middlesbrough was doing none of that.'

The traditional commitment to no compulsory redundancy and the desire to see Middlesbrough as the leading town in Teesside may have created the conditions for a budgetary crisis, but that does not explain why Middlesbrough management had not taken any measures to rectify the situation.

John's analysis implies the existence of a deficit in responsibility by the leadership in management:

> 'It was just then, of course, that having created this entity, nobody wanted to take the management or leadership responsibilities to do anything about it, and so month by month it simply got worse and bigger.'

On his arrival John decided that emergency actions were necessary to deal with the budgetary crisis. The problem was so bad that it was necessary to make people redundant, and people in management jobs in particular would have to lose their jobs.

Talking more generally about local government leadership, John stressed his belief in self-assessment and self-criticism. This belief appears to have been a by-product of his experiences of Comprehensive Performance Assessment (CPA). But arguably it can also be seen as a logical outgrowth of his belief in leaders taking responsibility for putting things right.

> 'I think the other thing that's really important, that emerged out of the CPA process which I'm very keen to use professionally within the organisation, is the importance of self-assessment. I think organisations should be capable of being self-assessing without being afraid of self-criticism. Those councils who were surprised, or claimed to be surprised, by their CPA judgements, whatever the arguments about the pros and cons of the process of CPA, were those who had no real understanding of what they were doing or how their services were performing.'

Getting and keeping political support

He had to have a conversation with the council's political leadership.

> 'When I arrived at the beginning of February, I had to sit down with the Senior Politicians and explain that "This is a serious problem, you can't ignore it in the way that you've ignored it this far. Essentially the Council is spending way above its means, which means that we are accruing bigger and bigger deficits, and which technically are illegal under local government regulations."

His plan was for emergency action to deal with the budgetary crisis – there was no time for further delay.

> 'My core message to them was that the situation was so bad that the normal mitigation and remediation strategies that we would normally employ had been used up, and that unfortunately they were going to be faced with a compulsory redundancy situation.'

This was a critical conversation. Would the politicians support emergency action to tackle the causes of the budgetary crisis?

> 'The outcome was that the Labour Leadership of the Council accepted the reality of the situation and stood by their decision that we needed to act.'

But not all the Labour councillors agreed.

> 'A sizeable minority of the Labour Group basically entered into internal opposition with its majority colleagues on the Council. But the two opposition parties, the Lib-Dems and the Conservatives, were broadly sympathetic to the idea that something needed to be done to address a worsening situation.'

The split in the Labour Group over this issue was encouraged by pre-existing differences. This is a view that John subscribed to:

'Some of their internal differences pre-dated my arrival. They were to do with personal rivalries, the fact that there had been a leadership challenge at the start of the new unitary, one faction had won, the other which had expected to win lost. They remained unhappy with the leadership and opposed them from within the group and local party. What happened in 1998/99 simply compounded the differences that existed within the majority group.'

The continued support of the senior Labour Party politicians in the majority group could not be taken for granted. John worked hard to maintain it:

'My work with the Politicians was to keep them robust about the need for the change, to keep them well informed. I spent hours and hours talking with them, explaining, answering questions about the position we were in and the way we could move forward.'

Looking back and with the benefit of hindsight, John regarded the sustained support of the politicians as the first success for the change process:

'The first success was the politicians in the majority holding their nerve on the matter.'

The new management team

John had been headhunted because changes were needed in management arrangements and he recruited a new top team of four corporate directors. They were all brought in from outside the organisation. It was to this team that John looked for his leadership group in bringing about changes.

'I arrived in the February, the new Corporate Directors started in May of that year, and between February and May I had brought them together on a couple of week-ends so that we could spend the time together thinking about the changes, me informing them about the difficulties about the budget, and what we were going to have to do about it.'

In the course of the first year John and his team put the new core structures in place. A traditional departmental structure had been created in 1995. John restructured the council into a small number of broad service groups (corporate services, education, environmental services, regeneration and housing, social care and health). Reflecting on this a few years later, he described the introduction of major senior management changes across the organisation as very successful.

Conflict with the unions

The main initial trade union response to John's emergency plan was outright opposition. Later on the trade unions offered some counter-proposals. John said that the union proposals were considered in detail, 'but we didn't find them workable or they only delayed the situation'. The decision to take emergency action and make people redundant was implemented in June 1998.

Public relations

As well as working with politicians and managers, John was meeting with the citizens of Middlesbrough. 'I spent a huge amount of time in 1998 and 1999 addressing public meetings across the town. I think I must have addressed at least a hundred public meetings.' These were big meetings.

> 'I don't think I ever addressed a meeting in that period of less than 100 people, but some of the meetings had as many as 400 or 500 people. So this was an amazing period, but also an amazing experience because, as a new Chief Executive and being new to the town, it was a fantastic way of learning about the area and getting to meet a lot of people, even if they didn't all agree with what we were doing or what we were saying.'

John held the view that when the problem was explained there was a good chance the public would side with the council rather than the trade unions.

> 'I took the view that in a town like Middlesbrough that had gone through years of major industrial change and restructuring, where there probably wasn't a family in the whole of the town that hadn't had a member who'd been made redundant either in the steel works or the ship yards or the chemical companies, that they were not likely to be hugely sympathetic to what the press and they might regard as Town Hall bureaucrats being made redundant. It was a tough judgement to make, but actually it proved to be absolutely correct because when the Trade Unions tried to make a town-wide campaign of this, they got absolutely no support at all, including from the newspapers.'

These public meetings were not about sharing a vision of a future. They were arguments and rows about what needed to be done to create the potential for a better future:

> 'Some of the meetings were incredibly vitriolic, but by and large I don't think there was a single occasion when I was unable to actually speak. Some of the sessions were very, very heated. Some individuals were very upset and very angry. There was lots of shouting going on, but I think on every occasion I managed to get my point across and also to answer lots of questions.'

Coping with personal attacks

Compulsory redundancy notices were issued in June of 1998. This was just within a few months of John's taking up the position of Chief Executive. This was not an easy time for John:

'You can imagine the atmosphere of the place was incredibly difficult and volatile. The Trade Unions obviously didn't like this. They were incredibly angry. They campaigned massively across the organisation and in the town, and they put huge pressure on the majority of Labour Councillors who had supported the change programme.'

John himself was a target.

'It was a very painful time for everybody. I was under immense pressure on a daily basis, I was being physically threatened and received many, many more threats. Obviously I didn't like having to do it and, of course, as the new Chief Executive being seen as the one who comes in to do this, was not what I would have preferred as my entry into the job. It became very personalised, I was regarded as the Hatchet Man from Tyneside because I had been previously working in North Tyneside and there were all sorts of rumours that I was deliberately brought down to butcher the organisation and to make people redundant and to deal with the left wing of the Trade Unions. It was all conspiracy theories fuelled and developed as part of a campaign of misinformation, but we had to deal with it. It was as rough a period in maintaining leadership, direction and focus as you're going to experience.'

Crisis as a platform for more change

Despite all the difficulties of 1998, the emergency action taken by John and his colleagues with the support of the politicians enabled the local authority to re-balance its finances. By March 1999 John was satisfied that the budgetary and financial changes he had instigated were beginning to bear fruit.

'In March '99 we were talking about introducing the Council's first three-year financial and policy programme and that provided us with a medium-term perspective. Many authorities were doing the same because Gordon Brown the Chancellor had introduced the three-year planning cycle and it was a sensible and obvious thing to do.'

The preparation of the budget for 1999/2000 took place on a more confident basis than had been possible a year earlier. The council prepared medium-term plans for improvement of services and introduced more changes and innovations.

'Those people who were made redundant had left the Council but there was still a lot of uncertainty around the organisation. New managers had arrived and most of the old management team had left. There were the beginnings of recognising a new way of doing things. We had also been working on new initiatives and projects. There were positive things that we were able to build upon – and that's what we started to do during 1999.'

John brought in a disciplined approach to the council's finances. In 2000 its balances were £9m. Middlesbrough Council consolidated reorganisation in 1999 and went on to continue making changes. These included work to forge 'a partnership between the key agency players across the district' and to move towards the creation of local strategic partnerships.

As already noted above, the council eventually came out of the Comprehensive Performance Assessment (CPA) in December (2002) as a highly regarded local authority. Evidently, the council's management and financial arrangements had been turned around over the 5 years John was Chief Executive.

Crisis and change: a multitude of actions at a multitude of levels

Sometimes books on strategic change present the realisation of strategic change as a highly programmed and sequenced event. It may be so, but the lived experience of crisis and turnaround for a leader may be best described as hectic and multi-faceted.

John summed up his first 2 years at Middlesbrough as 'So that was '98 and '99, I mean it was a massively hectic period'. Part of the explanation of this is the need for the managerial leader to engage with all the key stakeholders (politicians, public, managers, trade unions, voluntary and community organisations and so on). John, for example, spent a lot of time meeting people.

> 'It meant talking to all sorts of people and groups of course, not just the politicians and the public, but they were key folk. But I was spending a lot of time with the trade unions. I was spending a lot of time with managers, because obviously at the same time as trying to transform the budgetary situation I was having to transform the organisation.'

Part of the explanation in this case was also the need to make progress on different agendas. The council was trying to do four things simultaneously: deal with a budgetary crisis, reorganise management, address the democratic renewal agenda and improve services to citizens. While in this case study we have concentrated on the budgetary issue and, to a lesser extent, the management reorganisation, the third agenda was also important. In May 1999 Middlesbrough Council became one of the first to pilot an all-party cabinet and leader. It then went on to be one of the first UK councils to have a directly elected mayor.

A third part of the explanation, which is a similarity with another case study in this book (see the section on Wendy Thomson), is that the council was keen to volunteer for projects and programmes sponsored by the government. Middlesbrough Council was one of the first authorities that became an Education Action Zone. The council operated virtually all of the government's programmes: employment zones, health action zones, Objective 2, Sure Start, and SRB. This pattern of using government programmes benefited the council and citizens in terms of additional resources. But it also added to the furious pace of development and experimentation in the council.

Leadership at different levels

An interesting implication of all these changes and projects is the issue of who was responsible. John saw the responsibility for innovation in general as shared between innovators and leaders and occurring at many levels within the organisation. He referred to Belbin's concepts of management teams when explaining how innovators and leaders combined to bring about change.

'I think the innovators are not necessarily going to be the natural leaders. There are those in the organisation that come up with an idea; you then need other types in the organisation to test it out and see if it's worth pursuing; and then you need somebody within the organisation at some level who plays a leadership role and says "Right, to do this now we have to do this." So it requires a leadership action. Or, "We need to get the Council to formally agree this and take it forward." And that's about how ideas and management at different levels begin to take on slightly different qualities at a particular point, when to make it move requires a decisive action.'

In the following quote, John repeats and emphasises the point about leadership taking place at different levels:

'I think what I'm saying about innovation is that it can come from anywhere in the organisation. Anybody could be an innovator, anybody with a bright idea, but then it requires managers or leaders, or managers acting as leaders, to make it happen. The good idea, the innovation, stays a good idea if nobody is able to make it happen, and the making it happen must have, in my view, some leadership quality about it. It can be at a fairly low level. We're not talking here about the top of the tree all the time. Most of this leadership takes place at all different levels of the organisation. An organisation needs many leaders at different levels.'

The process for generating leadership at multiple levels was described by John as a process of cascading and this cascading was brought about by individuals, leaders demonstrating leadership. So managers learn leadership by observing leadership by those within the structure at the next level.

'A Chief Executive should know everything important to the authority that's going on in the organisation. But at an operational level you need effective managers. Organisations need to allow managers at all levels to use their judgement and make decisions. Corporate directors, as well as being effective managers, need also to demonstrate leadership within their remits, and so it goes on as you cascade it throughout the organisation.'

His explanation of leadership involvement in innovation centres on their risk-taking function. His type of leaders assume responsibility for the risk-taking:

'It might be argued that innovation in Local Government is actually not likely to happen without leaders, because innovation is the front end of change and it's the bit of change that might be more risky, and risk is not taken, I think, without leaders at various levels in an organisation. I think the two go together.'

A CASE STUDY OF WENDY THOMSON AT NEWHAM COUNCIL

Wendy Thomson joined the London Borough of Newham, a council in the East of London, in 1996. She was Chief Executive there until she left in 1999. During this time Newham Council became known for its bold improvements and for its role in piloting a new government policy known as 'best value'.

In the summer of 1997 the newly elected Labour Government announced it was going to replace compulsory competitive tendering by a new performance management regime, best value. This was intended to focus local government not only on performance and making improvements to performance, but also on making local government closer to the public it served. The new system, therefore, was to be built not only on performance indicators, regular internal review of all activities, and external inspections by an inspectorate, but also consultation of stakeholders, including the public, and best value performance plans that were to be presented to the public. In the early days it was expected that individual local authorities would develop local performance indicators to reflect local diversity, but in the event local authorities chose not to develop these and generally attention was mainly directed to the performance indicators set nationally. The system was also intended to encourage a pragmatic approach to keeping local government activities in-house; if better results for the public could be obtained by involving the private or voluntary sector, the local authority was expected to use these options. This aspect of best value was meant to be about putting the public first and was meant to reduce the ideological content of decision-making. This, and the requirements to consult the public and publish best value performance plans, represented a rethinking of the traditional social-democratic beliefs of welfare state society. If they worked, and thus if the public became a more influential voice in the design of local government services, it would have created a more democratic community and a less bureaucratic and less paternalistic local state. Arguably, the evolution in social-democratic beliefs was necessitated by the emerging post-industrial culture in society, which entailed a less work-centred outlook on life, weakening class loyalties in political voting behaviour, and increasing attention to consuming and life-styles. At the end of 1997 the new government released the news that Newham Council was to be one of a total of 34 pilot authorities, and one of four where best value was going to be piloted for the whole of the authority's services.

The council set itself very stretching goals for the pilot of best value. It wrote to the Department of the Environment, Transport and Region, in response to a consultation paper, that it was going to use best value to achieve in the course of 3 years:

- Overall cost savings of 5 per cent
- Improvement in service quality levels of 10 per cent
- A more pluralistic approach to service provision.

In 1999, when it was announced that Wendy was leaving the council, Andrew Foster, controller of the UK's Audit Commission, praised the council and commented on its 'outstanding record of improvement in public services with a citizen-centred approach' (*The MJ*, 4 June 1999: 3). Wendy confirmed that there had been a dramatic improvement in performance. She had monitored the council's performance using a basket of Audit Commission performance indicators. In 1996 Newham was 31st out of 33 London boroughs. Three years later, in 1999, when she left, it was 3rd.

There was evidence that the citizens of Newham were also more likely to rate it as a desirable place to live in 1999 as against 3 years earlier. It is unlikely that this was simply a reflection of the improvements in organisational performance. The council had also engaged with the business community and instigated improvements and developments in the area.

How had she done this in just 3 years?

Leading through strategic vision

When Wendy Thomson arrived in Newham Council as the new Chief Executive she embarked on a programme of visits with elected councillors to council wards. She used these visits to meet and talk to council staff. Some of the visits were unannounced, which could be alarming for staff, and which they apparently responded to with different degrees of enthusiasm.

The early result of these visits was that Wendy began to form an appreciation of how well the organisation was working and the direction in which it was going at that time. She commented on these visits, 'I learnt a lot.' She also discovered that those working in the Chief Executive's office had little knowledge of what was to be found in the wards she visited. This suggests that the top of the organisation – managerially and administratively – can become isolated from the front line of service delivery. She summed this situation up as a 'disconnect between the top office and what we actually did on the ground'. Far from the disconnection being seen as a problem, the isolation of the Chief Executive can be seen as normal. This was perhaps suggested by an assumption that members of the public who rang up the Chief Executive's office about services should be redirected to departmental managers that ran the services.

In Chapter 2 we looked at Bennis and Nanus's ideas about leadership that presented the leadership process as about, first, listening and asking questions and then, secondly, moving on to the formulation of a strategic vision. This means that leaders have to be good at listening, but then have to move towards taking up the responsibility of setting a direction for the organisation, which they can do by outlining a strategic vision. This further means that leaders have to both listen to the ideas of others and lead in formulating the vision. Moving from one activity to the other can at times require skill. Wendy Thomson followed the Bennis and Nanus model to the extent that she took time to speak, listen and learn and then she formulated a vision. In this sense she was acting as a visionary leader. We think the personal experience of movement through the process of visionary leadership – from listening to formulating a vision – was possibly the explanation of Wendy's observation that, 'It's a tricky thing between listening and leading.'

The vision she produced was an ambitious one. It did not centre on best value but on turning the area of Newham around. It had long been seen as a poor area of East London, a working-class area. In the 1990s only a very rare local authority Chief Executive would have imagined that it was possible to make anything other than very modest changes in the quality of life experiences in Newham. She did. This by itself singled her out as someone who was exceptional.

She came up with a vision that was based on thinking the unthinkable. Labour councils have tended to see themselves as the champions of the underdog, the protectors of the poor and weak. She had to think of the council's responsibilities in more inclusive terms. The council would have to care about the better-off as well as the poorer sections of the working class. She had realised that there were important social processes that reproduced the situation in Newham. In particular, she had realised that poor people tended to move to Newham but then moved out again if they started to prosper. 'It was a place poor people went to on the way to getting rich.' She had a simple proposition for turning around this situation. She thought that the council needed to adapt the area so that as communities and families improved their circumstances they chose to stay rather than leave.

Was her vision regressive? We would say it was the opposite. There is no necessary implication that the vision entailed a move away from solidarity and social justice, although it did indicate widening the net to include more sections of the community in social solidarity. *De facto*, a local authority defines the nature of social solidarity when it uses tax revenues to determine who will get services and get support. Back in the 1970s some councils tended to see social solidarity in terms of the (shrinking) manual working class. In Wendy's rethinking of the responsibilities of the local authority she was in effect thinking about widening social solidarity to include the members of Asian and other communities who kept on leaving Newham as soon as they could because of the housing and schooling that were available. 'If they made a decision to stay, then that area would transform itself, turn it around. And that became the strategy. So we wanted to keep them in the schools . . . [and ensure there were] bigger houses.' The end result of the strategy would be a more diverse and less uniform community in terms of economic composition. In other words, the local authority would see this as essential to a democratic community, that is, that it should address the needs of the many and not just the needy. These are not easy arguments to make and there is no doubt that the vision would be regarded very doubtfully by old-style social-democratic politics where the immediate objective is income and wealth equality and the state is seen as key in redistributing income and wealth to the manual working class.

She began drafting her ideas and discussed these with councillors in this draft form. Finally she prepared a statement of this vision in a paper called 'Putting Newham on the Map'. The paper set out an ambitious agenda for change and was aligned to the New Labour thinking, which was to form the agenda for reform in local government from 1997 onwards. It offered a new sense of strategic direction and a way out of simply calling for higher and higher spending on social services. She thinks there was a perception that this vision was her strategic vision. 'I think it was seen as my overall vision really, and I think people adopted it.' However, it was in fact a synthesis of Wendy's own ideas and the ideas of other people. It was based on what she had learned from all the people she had met. In her opinion: 'it had enough of others in it for it to be taken on board, I think.'

The elected councillors debated the vision and it was evident that there was no immediate universal acceptance. Some councillors had doubts. For others the vision statement was what they had been looking for. We might even guess that when Wendy was recruited it would have been obvious to the leading councillors what sort of contribution she could make. She provided the organisational expertise they needed to take their ideological agenda and make it a feasible proposition. The councillors had their own ideas, the paper recognised this, and helped to fill in some of the ideas that had been missing. Eventually a majority voted in favour and the strategy was adopted.

There were two other constituencies who mattered and to whom the vision had to be communicated. One of these was the private sector. The strategic vision of persuading people who became better-off to stay in Newham led to the idea that changing Newham had to have a physical dimension. This meant a significant amount of building in the docks and shopping centre developments. In consequence, a key issue for the strategy was the role of the business community as a key stakeholder, and the role of property developers in particular. Wendy was involved in targeting the business community, especially big property developers. Their role in bringing about physical changes in Newham was crucial.

The other key constituency was the employees of the council, especially professional employees. Communicating the vision to them and getting them to share it was not without challenges. We will return to this point later, but we note here Wendy's own reflections on the matter some years later. Looking back, Wendy said: 'I don't think there are many organisations where I'd do that again in that way ... I think times have changed ... those were the times when Labour was still becoming 'new' and people had to stand up and be "new". I don't think you need to be quite so heroic now . . .. But it had a downside in that we had to work hard to get ownership.'

Creating or stimulating the conditions for visionary leadership

Some of Wendy's actions and initiatives can be seen as creating conditions supportive of visionary leadership. For example, she was interested in HR development and Organisation Development to go alongside her work on strategy and performance management. She commissioned a top management development programme to coincide with the implementation of the vision.

> 'It was for 160 managers and it was based on multi-learning styles. There was an element of teaching; an element of project working to an actual budget that had to be done; and action learning. It was compulsory. People were assessed before it, and assessed after it, on skills – some quite basic skills like numeracy and literacy. They had to work on projects on topics they knew nothing about with colleagues they wouldn't normally work with.'

But much more striking in Wendy's account of the impressive changes occurring in Newham were the features of the experience that are not prominently theorised in accounts of visionary leadership (Bennis and Nanus 1985; Gabris *et al.* 2000). These are discussed in the next section.

What is left over?

Successful leaders such as Wendy do not operate only at the level of abstract ideas. A key feature of Wendy's account of her experiences as a leader during a period of substantial change and improvement was her emphasis on getting and understanding detailed information and knowledge. She thinks that it is critical for public services leaders to personally have a grasp of the detail. In the past she has advocated the use of service sampling, a process whereby top managers spend time in the front line of service delivery so they can directly observe and reflect on the concrete nature of services they manage. She still advocates its usefulness, because she thinks it provides top-level managers with the rich contextual understanding that they need.

Why this emphasis on information and detail? This may seem surprising if we stereotype leaders as visionaries or the people who dream the big dreams and inspire others to take these dreams and turn them into reality. However, case study research by Borins (1998: 157) suggested that successful public sector turnarounds occur where leaders not only create vision and inspire people but also know their business and know their key stakeholders well.

> 'They did . . . display an unusual ability to create vision and inspire others . . .. Their expertise in their business or their knowledge of the stakeholders appears to have been the critical factor.'

If successful leaders are good at the vision aspect of change, but also good at detail, is this a coincidence? Arguably, the attention to detail may be important for the feasibility of the visions that leaders espouse.

This attention to empirical detail came through strongly in the Newham approach to implementing best value. The council's Best Value Team created a Toolkit designed to ensure reviews of activities were based on very detailed analysis. This Toolkit guided managers through a process that entailed detailed descriptions of activities, resources, costs, consultation findings, and targets for performance quality improvements, cost reductions, and community and user perception improvements. It also provided for an analysis of suppliers and partners, performance and risk assessments, and process improvement priorities, and for the description of a delivery plan. The outline of the descriptions, assessments and plan was backed up in the Toolkit by 11 pages of guidance to managers to ensure that they got the information correctly detailed.

Wendy Thomson also emphasises the need for performance management systems to use 'live data' from operational systems (e.g. payroll data), not data that are specially compiled to make returns as part of a reporting system and are therefore likely to be old data. She also emphasises the need for these to be data that the managers are using to manage the organisation. The point, she argues, is to have data that are used, not data that are merely obtained for 'academic' understanding. She considers it important to invest time and effort in getting information systems right. This includes investing in IT systems that can help ensure the integrity of the data, their relevance and accuracy.

Leaders do not just communicate and inspire; they also argue and handle conflict. While there was no intense conflict and resistance to the strategic changes in Newham, there was some latent conflict and resistance. There was some resistance at the political level, although in overall terms the political support for the vision was strong. In the end the opponents were won over:

'Some people [councillors] voted against the vision, and when it went to Council itself it was really very emotional. The key people stood up and spoke for it, and one person had been holding out against it. By then it had been through lots of committees. It had been all round the Council. Then she stood up and spoke on behalf of it. For whatever reason, she decided that it was going to be a good vision.'

The vision was not popular with all members of staff. A council strategy of keeping the newly prosperous citizens in the borough inevitably was also a shift from concentrating on 'needy' people. Wendy responded to employee doubts about the strategy by trying to argue and convince them. This need to argue and persuade means the leader needs to have energy and be resilient:

'I argued . . .. Sometimes it's not very comfortable. Having an argument is not always a very comfortable thing to happen . . . once I think I've got it right in my head about what we should do, then I go ahead to try and persuade people.'

Obviously argument and persuasion can be a debate about actions and consequences and can lead to consensus. But sometimes argument can turn into rows and then even open conflict. There was substantial open conflict in the other two case studies in this chapter, but conflict on the same scale appears not to have materialised in Newham. But we should note Wendy's statement above that it was hard work getting the organisation to own the strategy.

Leaders such as Wendy do not just empower; they also plan. Wendy commented on her own close attention to planning.

'Personally I've probably enjoyed the strategy, representational, communi-cational side of the job [of Chief Executive] but I do also spend a lot of time going into quite a lot of detail of exactly what people have to do, when they have to do it, whether or not they've done it and making sure that they do it.'

This is an important point. Kotter (2001) and others have tried to draw a clear line between leadership action and management action. Leaders have strategies; managers plan. Wendy appears to cross over the boundary – being interested in planning as well as strategy. Moreover, she appeared to recognise the academic debate about these matters with the following recent observation:

'Leadership is [deciding] what you do. Management is [deciding] how you do it. And doing the right thing is part of what we need to deliver, and that does require a capacity of strategic thinking and an ability to organise that thinking into activities that can be undertaken.'

It should be noted that there was an expectation that Wendy would plan when she went to Newham Council. In fact, she agreed as a con-dition of her contract as the new Chief Executive of Newham that she would produce a plan at the end of her first 100 days. This can be seen as part of a pattern of macho leadership. She was not entirely happy with this. It was pressure to behave like a table-banging leader who 'comes in and says I'm going to change all that'. Whether this is ever a good way for a leader to behave is difficult to say, but it certainly has been a view in some times and some places about how strong leaders should behave. She did create a plan as required by her contract.

Leaders like Wendy do not merely hope for improvements; they also make use of performance management. Wendy viewed empowerment (a leadership process according to Kotter) as important; but she also thought performance management (a management process aimed at planning performance and controlling it) was important. Empowerment and performance management are not either-ors. A leader makes sure both happen.

> 'You don't just do empowerment. You don't just do performance management. You don't just do strategy. You recognise that these things are a set of activities that all need to be done.'

Judged by the amount of consideration Wendy gives performance management in reviewing her experiences of leadership, we are tempted to conclude that as a leader she has been just as concerned with performance management as she has been with empowerment. It is clear that she sees performance management systems pragmatically and is concerned to use them as a lever for moving the organisation forward.

She accepts that the performance measures they were using in Newham Council were not perfect from a technical point of view, but nevertheless she tried to make performance management meaningful at the personal level:

> 'So nothing was perfect. But if it was only half right we were counting in the right direction, and getting these numbers to move. I tried to get people to think of it not as a number, but the net effect of human endeavour. So that if you've got the Housing Benefit [numbers to] shift, [then it was because] thousands of people had done something different, altered their behaviours, the claimants were actually bringing the right paperwork through to us, [and we were] issuing the right amount of money in the right time-frame. So when you moved it [the performance indicator number], it wasn't just a technical issue, it was a personal issue. So when we went up to third overall [among the London boroughs], even if it wasn't technically right, it was hugely motivational and it was true that a lot of people had been trying to get the numbers to shift.'

It appears that making performance management work was far from effortless. Managers may resist; they may try to argue against the measures of performance or the data: 'these numbers aren't right, it's not my responsibility, it's someone else's fault, or there's nothing we can do about it now anyway.' The leader bringing in such a system has to be prepared for resistance. An experienced leader expects the arguments and rebuts them.

'You go through the pain threshold, you just wade your way through them [the arguments]. You just go through the bullshit until it's finished . . . . [W]hen they tell you the numbers are wrong, you think "Wow the numbers are wrong, go back and try and fix them up". But when I'd done it three times, they all knew I'd say that [they should go back and fix the numbers] . . . . Anyway, you go through all those arguments until it becomes ideologically and personally unacceptable not to know the numbers. And I would encourage people to put their numbers in the faces of their staff all the time . . . . So you'd have Housing Benefit staff with all the charts, and at the end of the week the Director would come down and write the trajectory for the next step, and if it went down, he'd sniff, and if it went up he'd be happy . . . with 14 offices they could get a league table that shows all 14 offices . . . . It got very personal.'

Another feature of the experience described by Wendy was that the radical improvement in performance was the result of a torrent of changes.

'We were also doing all those initiatives . . . . We weren't just running on the vision in abstraction. We had tons of urban regeneration money. We had every kind of action plan going. We had a huge drive on education achievement . . . . We were doing best value and we had to do it better than anybody, because we were like that. If there was anything going we had to win it. So there really [were] quite a lot [of initiatives] . . . there wasn't just one thing that was done. Everything was being done at once . . . actions on employment, actions on education . . .'

But we must set against the multitude of changes that occurred a unity of vision and purpose. As Wendy put it: 'We had inside clarity of purpose. A strategy.'

The final feature of her experience of leading change we think worth highlighting can be seen as harking back to the point made by Bennis and Nanus (1985) about the importance of energy. But it is given a special twist in the experience reported by Wendy. The change process may require raised energy levels within the organisation, but the leader also needs personal energy and, as a dimension of that personal energy, needs resilience. The need for personal energy and resilience may be linked to conflict and resistance centred on the changes the leader is making (Heifetz and Linsky 2002). An example of this is the introduction of a performance management system. This is naturally going to be an uncomfortable experience. Wendy understood this, 'But you have to continue doing it and not get guilty about upsetting people.'

But the change-related conflict is not the only conflict demanding of attention. Nor was it the only conflict expensive in terms of leadership energy. Wendy Thomson had to deal personally with two councillors whom she suspected of misconduct. In one case she suspected that there had been interference with the conduct of an election.

'Personally in that time I had a couple of Councillors . . .. I had to set up an enquiry and I did it before we had legislation . . . so personally as the Leader, the energy you need to do this is huge, and when you've got drains on it, that's hard.'

Of course, it may be that even these types of conflict are important for the eventual success of a leader seeking to bring about big change. A willingness to expend energy and deal with the consequent personal attacks made on the leader could be seen as important in signalling that the overall culture of the organisation was changing. This does not make handling the personal attacks easy to deal with: 'Personal abuse, privately, publicly, in every place you can – not just to me but to my staff.'

Leaders like Wendy need an inner strength that keeps them moving towards their goal of radical improvement. This seems to come from a belief in the importance of building public services that serve the public.

A CASE STUDY OF LEIGH LEWIS AT JOBCENTRE PLUS

In March 2000 the UK's Prime Minister, Tony Blair, announced the merger of the Benefits Agency and the Employment Service, saying that a new agency would provide an improved and integrated service to job seekers beginning in 2001. The new agency was to be responsible for providing information and services on job vacancies and a range of benefits (job seekers allowance, income support, incapacity benefit, severe disablement allowance, maternity benefit, widow's benefit, industrial injury disablement benefits, and invalid care allowance). David Blunkett, then the Employment Secretary, was quoted as saying that the government wanted 'one door to knock on' for people of working age (http://news.bbc.co.uk/1/low/uk_politics/679311.stm [downloaded 25 November 2003]).

This merger appears to have been more than a simple improvement in welfare services. It was also, it seems, an attempt to modernise a part of the welfare state. Alistair Darling, at the time the Social Security Secretary in the UK government, was reported to have said the government was moving from a 'passive' to an 'active' welfare system. Andrew Smith, a Labour Member of Parliament for Oxford East, in June 2002, welcomed the fact that Oxford was to get one of the new 'Jobcentre Plus' offices and commented on the help it would provide in moving people from welfare into work. The welfare state reform theme was also suggested by the MP's observation:

'Last week I went with the Prime Minister to talk to staff and customers at the Streatham "Jobcentre Plus" office in London. The central role of Jobcentre

Plus is moving towards a welfare state which helps individuals.'
(http://www.andrewsmithmp.org.uk/News_17June02_JobCentre.htm
[downloaded 25 November 2002]).

The union response to the merger announcement was reported as being a 'cautious welcome'. Mike King of the Public and Commercial Services Union was quoted as saying: 'We want any staff savings put into improving services' (http://news.bbc.co.uk/1/low/uk_politics/679311.stm [downloaded 25 November 2003]).

In fact the new agency, known as Jobcentre Plus, formally came into existence in April 2002. Its Chief Executive was Leigh Lewis. As a sign of the political importance being placed on leadership of government 'delivery businesses', the job of Chief Executive of Jobcentre Plus came with the status of Permanent Secretary. In the civil service world the Permanent Secretary of any government department is a hugely important and influential figure and even those at this level not in charge of a Department carry considerable authority.

Leigh Lewis came to this new job with experience of running the Employment Service. He had become the Chief Executive of the Employment Service just months before the May 1997 general election that resulted in a new Labour government. The new government had four credit card pledges to the electorate. One of them was the New Deal for Young People, a pledge to end long-term youth unemployment. The government asked the Employment Service to take the lead in delivering this part of the new agenda. Over the next five years Leigh led the top team of the Employment Service, 'and in that time I think the Employment Service had changed and had become a more customer-focused, more responsive, more welcoming organisation'.

While Leigh was leading the Employment Service, government ministers were beginning to think that the existing organisational separation of the job finding and the benefit payment processes was artificial and there was an idea of bringing together two separate services to form a new integrated organisation. The scale of this organisational change was huge. The Employment Service had employed 35,000 people, and in 2000–1 had information on 400,000 job vacancies. The Benefits Agency employed 70,000 people. (Note that the part of the Benefits Agency dealing with pensioners was spun off into a separate Pension Service, so only the part of the Benefits Agency that dealt with people of working age went into Jobcentre Plus.)

'As we got to the end of the present Government's first term I think that Welfare to Work policy was assuming ever larger importance . . ... And [there was] a belief that we had a compartmentalised system. For people who were unemployed we had a Job Finding and Benefit Payment Organisation – the Employment Service with a pro-active support role; it would help you pro-actively to overcome the barriers to getting to work. For the rest we had a more passive Benefit Payment Organisation – the Benefits Agency – whose job it was to pay out the money to which people were entitled. That's a very important job, but it didn't have such a pro-active role and had relatively little face-to-face contact with many of its customers. Increasingly [there was] a belief from Ministers that this was an artificial distinction, and that we needed a single government organisation which would have, for the whole range of welfare recipients of working age, two objectives: one was paying benefit of course to people who were entitled to it, but the other was pro-actively help-ing people to overcome barriers, to acquire skills to get into work, to be able to hold down and retain employment. And that was the philosophy behind Jobcentre Plus.'

The government decided to advertise for a Chief Executive of Jobcentre Plus. Leigh decided to apply: 'Because I shared the belief that this was the right thing to do, I went for it and got it.' This was in March 2001.

Success?

Two years later in 2003, when we spoke to Leigh, he had in fact just left Jobcentre Plus after 6½ years in this and his former role as Chief Executive of the Employment Service (he is now Permanent Secretary for Crime, Policing, Counter-Terrorism and Delivery at the Home Office). Even by then the change process was not yet complete but the pilot phase of opening 49 new integrated offices was over. By the mid-dle of 2003 there were about 300 integrated offices, well on the way towards the network of 1,000 new-style offices.

Leigh rated the changes as being successful. 'I think the concrete evidence is the organisation exists, it has palpably generated a new relationship with its customers, both individuals and its employers, and it's got very high customer service ratings.'

> 'And there's a whole set of ways in which Jobcentre Plus measures its cus-tomer satisfaction. Customer satisfaction with the new-style service is incred-ibly high, top 80s/low 90s in satisfaction ratings, almost unheard of for Government Agencies, it's hitting its targets in terms of people placed into work and help and back received payments. Employers, who are an incredi-bly important group of customers as well, because if Jobcentre Plus doesn't meet employer needs there are no jobs which it can offer to its customers, are high in, and growing, satisfaction levels as well. So, a lot of evidence that the organisation is winning, not losing. Not, to be clear, a perfect organisation, not without its problems.'

Strategic vision

Deutsch (1966) suggested that there were two types of leader in his studies of political communications and control. The first, prophetic leaders, were leaders in terms of new ideas, whereas the second type, continuing leaders, exercised the power that implemented ideas. Something similar to this appears to have occurred in the case of the vision for the new agency. As we have seen above, the idea of inte-grating the two services appears to have originated with government ministers. Leigh Lewis and his top team then picked up the political idea, developed it and tailored it. The embryonic statement of the vision for this new agency can be traced back to the Prime Minister and a statement he made to the House of Commons:

> 'In a sense there was a vision, the Prime Minister in I think March 2000 set out the vision, the Government's vision, there was a statement in the House of Commons as to why the Government was doing this and what it wanted to achieve. So that became the vision. But inevitably it was a pretty broad vision and it left a lot of the details still to be painted in and a lot of the detail to be worked through, and I guess that I saw one of my key early challenges when I took the job as trying to be able to make that vision meaningful to the person in Barnsley or Edinburgh because, in a sense, unless people through-out the organisation can to some degree share the vision then you are not really going to achieve it.'

Part of the work of developing the vision so it can be implemented involves discussion and a search for a formulation that is acceptable in the civil service. For leaders of reform this experience is in part defined by the fact that civil servants in different countries can have quite a col-legiate culture. The leaders of reform are seeking consensus and acceptance of the vision, and so in principle the idea of a collegiate consensus is not undesirable. But the pre-existing collegiate consensus can in some situations be a problem. It can impede modernisation. This occurs where the collegiate atmosphere works to make leadership too cautious (see Schacter 1994 on Paul Tellier's leadership of public services reforms in Ottawa). It is also apparent that new ideas have to run the gauntlet of competing interests and the complexities of over-lapping mandates that can degenerate into 'turf wars'. It is apparent that Leigh Lewis was able to work skilfully in and around the culture of collegiality and the plurality of departmental interests and man-dates to produce an acceptable vision. He also had to continue to pay attention to the other key stakeholders – the job seekers, employers and staff.

> 'The truth is that you operate in a complex world which is both collegiate and challenging at one and the same time, and out of a whole set of discussions came gradually more detailed iterations of the Prime Minister's vision and they started to be drawn down to a lower level. I had a lot of influence in that process, but it was not my process to control in its entirety. I had to ensure that a lot of other stakeholders were alongside me, that Ministers were comfort-able with the way we were articulating the Prime Minister's vision and so on. And there were a lot of people involved; first of all you have Government Departments with interests quite rightly to pursue and defend, so the interest of the Treasury is "Is this going to cost a lot of money, what are we going to get from it, how are we going to know we are succeeding, what are the out-comes going to be, what are the targets going to be, were they stretching enough, were they tough enough?" You had the Secretaries of State most directly concerned wanting to be sure that the policy outcomes and objectives were the ones they wanted to achieve and not some group of objectives that

belonged to somebody else, and it's not impossible of course in any Government system, that different departments have different competing priorities. And then you had a set of other stakeholders, stakeholders representing the staff, stakeholders representing the customers, stakeholders representing employers, etc., and again part of the challenge is to try and emerge with a vision and a way ahead and structures which command the confidence of the widest possible group of the people you are trying to work with, and it's not an easy process.'

So, summing up, we should note here three things about the strategic vision. First, the kernel of the vision came from the Prime Minister, the most senior political leader in the government. Second, the detailing of the vision was done in a way that made it acceptable to other stakeholders, both within the organisation and at a political level. We might think of this as being a process of completing the vision to make it meaningful and acceptable to those who have to implement it and those key suppliers of political support. Thirdly, there were discussions with various stakeholders but these were not really part of the search for a vision so much as part of this process of completing it.

Management team and the Board

Leigh was leading strategic change based on the vision, and was anxious to stress the importance of the top team in having made a reality of Jobcentre Plus, but on the day he was appointed he was almost literally the only person in this new agency. He therefore had no top management team. He had no board. He had no organisational structure. He would soon have to handle the building of a new organisation from two existing ones. He was one man by himself and soon he would be merging two organisations with 100,000 people and creating a new integrated organisation with 1,000 offices. The endeavour was also quite unusual in the civil service – to create a single integrated service with a new culture that was customer-focused. The change could not be programmed. It had to be developed. 'There was no road map, and there was no script, so we were making a lot of it up as we went along.'

He had to work on several fronts at once. He could not simply concentrate on communicating the vision. He also began, at the same time, 'to put in place some of those basic building blocks that no organisation can exist without, a top team, a structure, a vision, objectives, budgets – you name it we didn't have it, and those were the immediate priorities'.

He needed a top management team. 'I began assembling my top team because you simply cannot do this yourself.' That was his first, and key, priority.

He needed a new board. This was an opportunity to open up thinking by bringing in some new perspectives. It was also important to begin integrating the organisation and thus avoiding a composition based on simply the former services.

'The make up of the Board was important. We needed to have a balance between the two former organisations, a balance of skills. But I was also keen to bring in some people from outside as well, and we did that. So we had a mixture ... appointments were made of people from the former Employment Service and the Benefits Agency, but we also brought in three Directors effectively from outside, and that was important to do . . .. Two from the private sector, and one who had actually been for a period in the Employment Service from an NHS Trust, where she had achieved a great deal. The three people we brought in, one was the Chief Operating Officer, in effect my Deputy; one was our HR Director who came in from a banking and retailing background, and one was our Director of Employer Services who came from a sales and marketing background . . .. That did a number of things – firstly, it stopped people, even within that Board, falling back into tribes or camps, because it wasn't just "we're from the Employment Service, we're from the Benefits Agency." Secondly, it brought in a set of different perspectives as well, so that there were people prepared to say "Yes, but hang on, we don't have to do it like that, nobody's written that in tablets of stone, why don't we do it like this, why don't we think of . . ." so it changed the dynamics.'

Communicating the vision to staff

Communicating the vision of the future for this new organisation was not expected to be easy. It looked a tough job to the new Chief Executive. Part of the problem was likely to be the atmosphere created by the announced merger. Groups of staff might, for example, feel they were being taken over rather than merged. Then there was the question of how each individual would be personally affected – would they win or lose out personally?

'There was quite a lot of background, quite a lot of baggage – these two organisations which were being brought together, had worked pretty well, had rubbed along at an operational level, and day-to-day contacts at working level had been pretty good. But there hadn't been a huge amount of shared agenda at senior level, and there was some mutual suspicion.

In certain respects there were operational requirements for the two to work together so they did, but it was relatively limited. There had been always joint groups, etc., but relatively limited. But there was also some suspicion in areas of both organisations. You can always parody these things, [but] many people in both of the two organisations thought they were being taken over by the other one because the agenda seemed to be about the work of one organisation and not the other. The person they had just appointed as Chief Executive of this new body had headed up one of the previous organisations and so on and so forth. Therefore, there were lots of fears, concerns, worries, anxieties, etc., and you can add to that all the normal myriad set of anxieties that people have when their future is uncertain. It's easy for us to say – well we're going to merge this organisation and that organisation. What most people would think about is not – "Is this a great idea in theory, is this going to be better for the future of the world" but "What's it going to mean for me?" because that's where people come from. So there were getting on for a hundred thousand people saying "What's this going to mean for me?" with all the uncertainty.

Some of our first steps therefore were trying to begin to paint a vision for the people of what this new organisation might be like, could be like, how it might be better for its customers and for them . . .'

As the quote underlines, a vision is not announced in a vacuum and staff evaluate the impact of the vision on their self-interests. This evaluation by staff is also surrounded, in this case at least, by staff anxieties relating to uncertainty.

So the challenge for the leader becomes how can you communicate the vision in the context of self-interest, anxiety and even suspicion when what you are seeking to do is get staff to think about the vision and ideally to become enthusiastic about what might be achieved. In other words, Leigh and his top team were hoping to inspire people to work for the vision's realisation. This was done not by the formal structures alone, but also by talking to people, by informal discussions and informal meetings.

'There are of course formal structures, so there were steering groups over-seeing the creation of Jobcentre Plus, there were ministerial meetings, etc. That was the formal part of the machine. There were an awful lot of informal discussions, meetings, consultations. One of my strongest personal beliefs as a leader in the public service, is that you have to get out there and talk to people . . .. So it was really important for us to get out there on the streets and start talking about this organisation, beginning to explain it, beginning to try to get people to buy in and people's appreciation, people's enthusiasm, to get people to look up from "Will I still have a car park space?" to "Hey, we might just be able to deliver something really good here".'

The pilot phase

Leigh was appointed in March 2001 and Jobcentre Plus formally came into existence in April 2002. The intervening period was used to pilot the concept of new integrated offices.

'Ministers had set us an objective, a very hard-edged objective. Ministers said that they wanted to have 50 new-style Jobcentre Plus integrated offices open and on the ground in October [2001], in just six months. So alongside all the rest we were actually seeking to get 50 completely different offices in place, operating with trained staff in a new way in six months flat.'

Since he had only been appointed in March 2001 this was a very ambitious objective.

'My reaction was that it was well nigh impossible, and so it proved, we only opened 49! One got away. Yes, it was a significant achievement, and it was interesting actually because, as I've occasionally said, the job of a Chief Executive, or anyone in a leadership role, is to be reasonably unreasonable. You have to press and set a challenge that is probably just past the edge of what most people think can be done. If it is so far past that edge as to be completely wild and utterly unachievable, then it becomes counterproductive. But equally you've got to keep pushing people to achieve that bit more than they thought they could achieve, and it became an incredibly powerful motivator – we were going to get those 50 offices open in October come hell or high water, and we got 49 of them open.'

Everything had to be done at a very fast pace. For example, the 50 offices were in 17 geographical areas, and each area was to have a manager. The process of drawing up job descriptions, person specifications, advertising, and then recruiting managers takes most public services organisations a long time. Leigh Lewis did not have a long time available:

'We advertised those jobs, which was one of the very first things we did because without key people to begin to lead a team in each area, there was no chance. And we carried out the interviews on a Thursday, and we made our appointments on the Friday, and people started their new roles on the Monday. I had simply said: "These are the terms of trade here. If you apply you will be starting work within 48 hours of your appointment."'

When people reacted by saying it was impossible, Leigh told them he was sticking to his timetable.

'I said, well, there you are, we're doing it. I don't want you to think you are talking to somebody unbelievably arrogant who thinks that the views of colleagues are of no consequence, but there are times, however, when you just have to say "I've been given the authority, I've been given the challenge, and I'm just going to use the authority and have the confidence to deliver what I need."'

Under the right conditions, working to a deadline can become highly motivating. And it is possible to tap into this by highlighting the challenge of working to short time-scales.

'The other thing we did which was fascinating, we had a countdown in days, the number of days that remained, working days to the date in October when these offices were due to go live. And it was an incredible motivator. You'd be sitting in a meeting having a discussion and you would say, this is a really interesting discussion, but there are 53 days left so what about taking a decision? And it became a huge motivator.'

In this first six months Leigh pushed people to achieve this ambitious target of opening 50 new integrated offices under a massive time pressure. It seems that for some people, anyway, this was motivating and thus energising.

Leigh regarded the pilot phase as important:

'Yes, it was a very important milestone because, at that point, we actually had Jobcentre Plus in existence. We actually had real offices and that was our first stage of the Business Plan. We had real staff in completely new-look offices . . .. We had people doing jobs in a completely different way, etc.'

The pilots were important because Jobcentre Plus as an organisation was learning what it had to do and because it powerfully demonstrated that it was possible to make rapid change successfully. Leigh saw both these things as important. He emphasised the demonstration aspect as particularly important. 'It was putting on a visible demonstration that this organisation now had a physical reality, was not just a piece of theory, and it was also a very tangible demonstration that we could operate in a very different way to different time-scales.'

Becoming a national organisation

With the pilot phase over successfully, 'the next challenge was to launch Jobcentre Plus as a national organisation'. That happened in April 2002.

On the new organisation's very first day, the very first Jobcentre Plus Business Plan was released. It covered the single year 2002–3.

'We wanted it to be in simple words with big pictures, bold pictures, and we had a very simple slogan that we worked up, "The job you want, the help you need" and really tried to set out what we were doing. Soon afterwards we produced our first ever vision document in the same style . . .'

In the 2002–3 Business Plan for Jobcentre Plus, Leigh Lewis set the scene as follows (p. 3):

'We are a brand new business within a very new Department: the Department for Work and Pensions. Our aim is to build an organisation that is dynamic, responsive and in tune with our customers' needs. The ambition set for us by Government – to transform what has too often been a passive welfare state, into a more proactive, individual and work focused service – is hugely challenging and very exciting.'

The idea of the new service was partly to promote work as the best form of welfare and therefore to help more people into work, helping them to move from being unemployed to being employed. At the same time, Jobcentre Plus would be treating people more like valued customers than passive clients. This meant paying attention to service standards and accessibility of the services offered.

Table 6.1 Active welfare.

	Bureaucratic service	Modern service delivery
Clients dependent on benefits		
Customers who have more independence (by working)		

Subsequently, in the document setting out the strategic vision for Jobcentre Plus, and associated plans, for the period from 2002 until 2006, it was envisaged that over the four years from early 2002 some 1,000 new integrated offices would be opened.

2001–2	56 pathfinder offices opened
2002–3	225 integrated offices opened
2003–4	250 integrated offices opened
2004–5	25 per cent of total integrated offices opened
2005–6	remaining integrated offices opened

But even before the arrival of 2002 there were ominous signs for the future of the strategic plan. The plan began to encounter resistance even at the pilot stage.

'When the 49 new offices opened on 22 October 2001 they were faced with strike action called by the main Civil Service Trade Union (the Public and Commercial Services Union – PCS) and the PCS called out all its members in those offices on strike on the day those offices opened. The issue was not about money, or terms and conditions of employment, it was about safety – screens.'

This was not the first time in the history of UK public services that there were disagreements between trade unions and employers about the use of screens to separate public service employees from members of the public. Screens can be an important physical protection for staff. The problem was that screens are seen as detracting from the service by politicians and managers wanting to create a stronger ethos of customer service, whereas trade unions see it as a health and safety issue in the sense that screens can protect their members from attacks by members of the public.

'Because one thing which we believed implicitly (and so did our ministers) was that if Jobcentre Plus was going to be a very different organisation in terms of the service it offered, it could not conceivably deal with its normal day-to-day customers behind a screen. Everyone will have their own views on this, but I do not believe I could try, in any real sense, to influence you or help you to think about your career, etc., if there was a large screen running between us. It is a huge psychological barrier. It sends the wrong messages out. Former Social Security Offices that had not been lavished with investment, were pretty grim places in many cases. They were not places you would want to stay in for any length of time. A single parent with a child would not have wanted to go into that environment. So we were pretty clear that we thought that Jobcentre Plus had to be a predominantly unscreened environment.'

This is not to say that there was no basis to the trade union concern. Members of the public have at times attacked public services employees.

'We were not uncaring about health and safety. The health and safety issues were very real because Jobcentre Plus deals with millions of people every week, and some of those people it has to say no to, no you're not entitled, no we don't think you are obtaining this money lawfully, etc. So you're not always giving welcome news or saying welcome things, and there was a real concern amongst some of our staff that it could not possibly be safe to do this job and to assess benefits, to give benefit decisions, in an unscreened environment. And without going back over the whole history, we had a trade union, which was quite political in its approach, and our belief based on a huge amount of evidence from this country and abroad, was that fundamentally the better you treat people, the better they respond, overwhelming evidence that if you treat people as human beings then they respond as human beings, though we went to great lengths to ensure that within that predominantly open plan environment, unscreened environment, we had safety built in. So in many of our offices we had security guards, we had closed circuit TV, we had our staff trained in handling difficult customers and difficult situations, we had panic buttons and alarms, etc.'

In December 2001 there was a national strike about the system of open plan working in the new offices. Mark Serwotka, the Public and Commercial Services Union (PCS)'s general secretary elect, was quoted as saying 'Opening unsafe Jobcentre Plus offices is gambling with the safety of staff' (http://news.bbc.co.uk/1/low/england/1759249 [downloaded 25 November 2003]).

According to Leigh this became the longest and toughest dispute in recent civil service history. While it lasted almost six months, it ended up with the union having to accept that the government was going ahead with Jobcentre Plus offices for the new agency in a predominantly unscreened environment.

CONCLUSIONS

In Chapter 2 we spent a lot of time looking at the idea of leadership as it is often portrayed these days – leaders made sure there is a strategic vision and they communicate it to inspire and empower managers and employees to deliver the vision. Does this conventional picture now look very one-dimensional? We think it does. First, the idea that leaders are primarily concerned with the vision and direction of the organisation and leave it to others to know the business in detail and think through action and implement appears to be wrong, certainly in respect of the experiences of Wendy Thomson while at Newham Council. She made sure she knew the operational side of the council's activities and stressed the importance of attention to detail. We saw in the case study of Wendy Thomson that she decided to carry out a detailed study of the activities of the council. She did not approach this through a desk exercise. She chose to visit each area with the local councillor for that area. Together with them she evaluated where the organisation was.

Secondly, the idea that leaders act in a straightforwardly organisational way misses out the organisation's political aspects. Not least among the political aspects is the need for political skills that leaders use in managing their relationships with elected politicians. As Moore (1995: 22–3) expresses it, managers in the public sector are involved in 'managing upward, toward politics, to invest their purposes with legitimacy and support'. Consequently, managerial leaders in the public services have to manage their relationship with politicians. This relationship transmits political risks as well as the usual risks of change failing. While we have already noted Heifetz and Linsky's point that adaptive change is experimental, the manager who experiments and fails can expect to be criticised by politicians and the media for wasting public money and taking chances. The managerial leaders in our cases did not fail.

We will recap some of the use of political skills in two of our three cases. In the first case, John Foster at Middlesbrough Council, our leader was in a difficult political situation when he first arrived. It was relatively easy for him to admit that there was a problem because he was not responsible for it. In contrast, the councillors that had appointed him were to some degree responsible for the problem. Would they admit it? John Foster demonstrated political skills by making it a top priority to meet with the leading councillors, get their recognition of the size of the financial problem, and check that he had their support for tackling it. This may sound obvious with hindsight and may sound easy to do. But the difficulties of what he did should not be underestimated. Leaders of organisations that have legally been responsible for the creation of serious problems do not find it easy to take the responsibility. He managed to get them to an acceptance of their responsibility, and without it, it is doubtful whether he would have been successful.

He also displayed political skills in sustaining the acceptance of the problem and the necessity for a solution. The council had to make cuts in the labour costs. Inevitably in a highly unionised public sector, this encountered major union resistance because complete job security could no longer be delivered. The leading party in the council was a social-democratic political party and hence had close links with the

public service trade unions. So it was important that the political leadership in the council was prepared for the real conflict of interest over
job security. In this case, the elected politicians in supporting his proposals were preparing the organisation for the necessity of change.
Because of these political skills he had the platform to appoint his own
top management team and make dramatic improvements in the
organisation as shown by a subsequent Comprehensive Performance
Assessment of the council. He took responsibility for leading the
process, but also ensured that the rest of the political and managerial
leadership shared that responsibility so he could not be politically or
organisationally outflanked.

In the second case Wendy Thomson, the new Chief Executive, had
a group of elected politicians who were keen to become a part of the
national approach to the modernising of public services. They were
critical of the present state of affairs. They had aspirations in respect
of the future. They lacked, however, the organisational knowledge
and expertise to formulate a vision for the council. They should not be
condemned for this. Elected politicians develop an essentially ideological relationship to change. They develop their ideas and agenda for
change through debates and deliberation within their political party, or
they develop them as they take part in electoral politics. But their
material experiences rarely foster expertise in influencing and intervening in the organisational activities of the public services. They are
of necessity reliant on organisational leaders to turn their political
ideas into something that delivers not just ideology but the modernised
services they want.

One example of her political skills was the way she visited local
areas with the councillor representing that area. Local councillors are
both representatives and members of the council. In the former role
they represent their local wards. The citizens in the local area may be,
and often are, dissatisfied with the current quality of services.
Therefore as a local representative the councillor should be acting as a
catalyst for change. In the role of council member they may be part of
the governing party. Therefore, as a member of the council, and therefore implicated in the service decisions made in the council, they may
feel a responsibility to defend them. This second role makes them
defensive and resistant to change.

Wendy Thomson, as the new Chief Executive, needed to encourage
among the ruling group of politicians sufficient criticism of their past
activities, in order to obtain a mandate for a new vision and for
change. By spending time with the councillors in the small locality that
they were responsible for, then it was much more likely that they
would, openly in her direct presence, be critical of what the council
actually delivered as public services. Subsequently, in the middle of
change, she could remind the elected councillors that the citizens in
their locality felt dissatisfaction with services. In other words, she was
able, if she needed, to reinforce their awareness of their representative
role and maintain their support for reform. So the fact of making the

visits to local areas with local councillors can be seen as political skills in action, using democracy to underline the responsibilities of elected politicians for reforming and improving local services.

As well as political skills in managing the relationships with elected politicians, there are also political skills in managing conflict. In the Jobcentre case, Leigh Lewis brought about the new activities and the new organisation that the politicians had envisaged. He turned their ideas into action. He did this despite considerable union resistance to new ways of working in the new agency. In fact, rapid development of the new service was achieved despite union resistance. His political skills as a leader involved him in finding a way of achieving his aims on the customer care front while making adjustments to ensure more security for staff.

Political skills in respect of conflict may include persuading and convincing people. While visionary figures may be known for their speeches and statements of the vision, leaders in a public services setting may be working hard to break down resistance to change by arguing and seeking to convince managers and employees of the rightness of the vision. At times, arguments may turn into rows and then conflict rather than consensus.

Political skills are needed to manage the process of taking people out of their comfort zones. While public services leaders may want to empower their managers and employees, they also take them into uncomfortable territory and demand and encourage them to increase productivity and innovation. This means raising the political temperature of the organisation and getting people into what Heifetz and Linsky (2002: 110) call a productive range of distress. 'You need to take the temperature of the group constantly, trying to keep it high enough to motivate people, but not so high that it paralyses them.'

Because of the political aspects of their work, public services leaders are attacked and criticised. They, therefore, also need personal energy and resilience to deal with problems that may not immediately seem to be related to the strategic change agenda, although there may be less obvious linkages to the final success of the leader.

Table 6.2 Successful leaders.

Not only . . .	But also. . .
Listening and asking	Arguing, debating and rowing
Formulating a vision	
Communicating and sharing vision	Concern for empirical detail
Communication skills	Planning actions in detail
Inspiring	Political skills
Empowerment	Managing conflict
Translating vision into reality	Performance management
Raising energy levels	Multitude of actions
	Personal energy and resilience

What is the implication of these case studies for our understanding of leadership in the public services? Arguably, writers such as John Kotter (2001), in seeking to get us to take leadership seriously, have contrasted it with management and offered us two ideal-type descriptions of these as distinctive systems of action. On the basis of the case studies above his representation of successful leadership may be too simplistic for that found in the public services.

CHAPTER 7

LEADING ORGANISATIONAL CHANGE AND RENEWAL? LIVERPOOL CITY COUNCIL

'Three years ago – would anyone have considered coming to ask Liverpool City Council for advice on anything?'

In our previous section we considered the way in which three case study scenarios, examples of what we term *adaptive leadership*, could be examined. In this chapter, we move one stage further on the journey towards an examination of our theme of new public leadership, and examine an organisation which in both operational and reputational terms, could be said to be as far away from the concept of renewal introduced in this book, as it is possible to be. Here we have the opportunity to consider the themes of redemption and renewal within a public service setting.

The question posed above, at the outset of this chapter, by a manager interviewed as part of this case study analysis of a major UK public service organisation, reveals the scale and scope of transformation which has been enacted within a relatively short time period. As we shall discover, the 'Liverpool miracle' represents a plausible example of how a complex and troubled organisation has arguably moved beyond a traditional change-focused agenda and into an area where it is possible to characterise the dynamic created as being one of genuine transformation and potentially sustainable renewal.

Located in the north-west of England, Liverpool City Council can be characterised as a large urban provider of local government services, employing approximately 19,000 people and with a budget in 2004/5 in the region of £1.2 billion. Its remit is diverse and includes education and social services, housing and allied benefits, as well as libraries, fire services and refuse removal. Such services feed in to executive portfolios that report to a Cabinet style of elected representation which has so far eschewed the increasingly popular tendency in the UK towards electing an individual into mayoral office.

Drawing upon the council's own documentation it is possible to see that as an organisation they are both reflective and pragmatic in terms of the journey they have undertaken, such that they state that:

'Historically Liverpool City Council had a reputation for bureaucracy, providing poor services, having little actionable knowledge on which to make informed decisions linked with one of the highest council tax rates in the country. The Council had developed its systems, processes and procedures for its own convenience and not for that of the customer.

However, all this has changed in just three short years with Liverpool becoming a leading customer centric authority. This dramatic change has been brought about in no small part by its customer service strategy and the willingness of staff at all levels to ensure that the strategy succeeds. The strategy is being implemented on a holistic rather than incremental basis and so encompasses both front line and back office environments. The City has moved away from providing access to services through the traditional functional boundaries at locations determined solely by the service provider.

We now:

- Place our customers at the heart of our organisation;
- Strive to achieve true first point of contact resolution (currently 85% and have empowered staff to take ownership for resolution);
- Have increased accessibility (both physically and through availability);
- Have gained a deeper appreciation of our customers, their differing needs, concerns and desires through research and converted this into actionable knowledge for improvements;
- Have also used this actionable knowledge to achieve intelligence-led local government that is driving strategy and structure;
- Continually challenge what we do and how we do it. Followed by a robust programme of continuous development and improvement;
- Have developed access channels around all forms of contact including face to face, telephony and electronic both reactively and proactively;
- Have developed the reach and richness of service delivery and included the ability to deal with complex and multiple requests;
- Have embraced the Government's objective of 100% of services being available electronically by 2005 (our aim is 2004 and we are on course to achieve this);
- Use technology to help and assist all members of the diverse communities that Liverpool serves.'

(Liverpool City Council 2003)

The extent to which leadership can be said to have been critical in driving forward such an apparently profound change agenda is the focus of this chapter. It is important to both note and commend at the outset, the impressive levels of co-operation that the council provided to this study of their organisation, coupled with the extent to which participants were willing to share their views and perceptions in an honest and open manner. In the authors' view it can really only be through such willingness to undergo external independent analysis, that real lessons in leadership can hope to be tested and shared.

THE LEGACY OF HISTORY

The 'reputation' that the council itself refers to, represents a history and culture that grew over some 300 years, embodying great cultural diversity; spells of economic growth and more latterly of decline. As a major port Liverpool was a centre for the import and export of both people and goods up to the end of the 1960s. Industries that had grown around this strategic link were likewise buoyant over a considerable and sustained time period.

Politically it is tempting to characterise Liverpool as being analogous to many American cities, where political leadership and representation appear almost the inviolable historical right of one party. However, to make such a characterisation in respect of Liverpool would be wholly wrong. In the 1950s the council was controlled by the Conservative Party; for much of the 1960s and 1970s it was Liberal and by the 1980s, the time of sharpest economic decline, the Labour Party had gained control. Analysing this trajectory of changing political influence may challenge the perceptions of many who know only of Liverpool through its media coverage from the 1980s onwards, when the Labour administration became a by-word for extremism. Yet this is to ignore the reality of Liverpool's historical development which perhaps owed rather more to free market enterprise theories than almost any other city in the United Kingdom. Quite simply, the influence of the docks as the key local employer, where employment, until the 1960s, was casualised, was potent in setting out a political environment which was far less polarised than is the case in other United Kingdom cities such as Sheffield, for example.

However, it remains true even today, that for many in the UK their views of Liverpool as an entity were formed and remain shaped by the legacy of a Labour administration which 'evolved' during the 1980s. Under the leadership of Derek Hatton, Liverpool as a local government entity appeared intent upon challenging almost every aspect of the Thatcher reformist agenda. As social and economic historians will attest, the costs and legacy of conflict are always high, and for Liverpool setting aside the damage done to reputation and confidence, the financial costs were immense in terms of undeclared and unmanageable budget deficits. Speaking at the time Neil Kinnock, the then leader of the Labour Party, sought to disassociate himself and the wider Labour movement from the extremist agenda of the Liverpool City Council administration:

'I'll tell you what happens with impossible promises. You start with far-fetched resolutions. They are then pickled into rigid dogma, a code, and you end in the grotesque chaos of a Labour council – a Labour council – hiring taxis to scuttle around a city handing out redundancy notices to its own workers.'

(Kilfoyle and Parker 2000: 87)

The perspective of one long-term employee on this situation provides invaluable context as to how the journey towards achieving change was set in motion:

'Quite simply even the loyal Liverpool electorate got fed up with paying for the Hatton legacy – the Liberal Democrats seized this opportunity in 1999 and brought with it their determination to put into practice a new vision for Liverpool, gaining overall control meant that new ideas actually had some authority behind them.'

1999 AND ALL THAT . . .

David Henshaw's arrival into the CEO role at Liverpool represented something of a homecoming for a 'local boy' who had already earned a reputation as an innovative and success-orientated local government senior manager. Born and educated in the Liverpool area, one should not underestimate the important message that his appointment sent out to the staff of the council and to the wider constituency of service users. Someone who was local and who both knew and understood the very particular Liverpool context was willing to take on the challenge of moving the council forward.

Whilst we shall discuss the personal leadership style and input made by Henshaw in some detail during the course of this chapter, it is important to recognise the scope and scale of what he and the organisation he led were able to achieve in a relatively short time-scale. In previous chapters we have discussed the increasingly important role of external performance review and here it is important once more to make reference to these processes. In Chapter 6 the results of a review process referred to as Comprehensive Performance Assessment (CPA) were used to establish that improvements in a local authority had occurred. The CPA analyses and assesses a range of data and performance indicators in order to provide a statement about an organisation's performance, achievement of value for citizens as well as capacity to innovate and drive forward change – the latter usually being referred to as Corporate Assessment. If we consider the outcomes of the Corporate Assessment review for Liverpool carried out in 2002, effectively only 2 years in to the development of the City Council under Henshaw, then one can see that there may indeed be valuable lessons to learn from questioning what underpins the 'Liverpool Miracle'.

'Liverpool City Council has a powerful, compelling and ambitious vision for improvement which has been communicated successfully to a wide range of stakeholders. Its clear aim is to transcend its past failures and become a flourishing and dynamic organisation which delivers high quality services and better quality of life for its citizens, within the context of a thriving city.

The approach which it has taken initially, in order to establish a sound basis upon which to build future improvement, has been characterised by a direct management style. This has been effective in launching the change process. The council is aware that the next stage in its progress will entail a move to a more consensual management style, greater empowerment of staff at all levels and the development of further detailed longer-term planning to supplement the growing accountability framework.

The council has strong leadership and good relationships between councillors and officers. Business process re-engineering has been used to increase efficiency and customer focus. The council has regained civic leadership and used partnerships and joint ventures to expand its capacity and raise the city's profile. However, although there are well-motivated and empowered staff at the top of the organisation and in some service areas, this is not reflected through all parts of the council . . .

The council is very committed to a performance management culture and a useful performance management framework has been introduced. There is clear corporate focus on performance indicators as a vehicle for improvement . . .

Over the last three years there have been measurable and significant improvements in the level and quality of service provided on behalf of the council in most priority service areas . . .

Liverpool City Council shows many of the characteristics of a learning organisation. It is self-aware and recognises the environment it is working in and the challenges it faces.'

(Audit Commission 2002: 4–5)

Clearly emerging from this review are issues of some major importance for any study of leadership – perhaps most critical being the reference to the highly directional style of leadership which the reviewers considered as being understandable given the particular context of the council but which they signalled would need to demonstrate itself to be capable of adaptation over the longer term. Perhaps the second key message emanating from this analysis is that of permeation of the messages around delivering a new type of service. Clearly one of Henshaw's key early challenges was to recruit a top team around him, into reorganised and refocused roles which would give momentum to service transformation plans. However, as we may recall from our discussions of the capacity for organisations to move beyond a change agenda and into the rather more sustainable waters of renewal, for this to happen requires that some level of understanding and ownership over both personal and organisational future direction, is shared across all strata. Certainly what the Audit Commission was flagging in 2002, was high degrees of commendable performance around instigating major changes; however, over the longer term, a renewal agenda had still to embed.

PASSING THE BATON – LIVERPOOL DIRECT

One of Henshaw's key principles as a public service leader would appear to stem from a deeply rooted belief that a range of providers should be capable of working co-operatively in order to achieve beneficial outcomes for all stakeholders. Certainly analysis of key activities and discussions with staff located across the complex and diverse organisation, indicated that the concept of partnership working was clearly understood as an organisational imperative – albeit that the mechanics of enacting such practices were, in reality, often fraught with difficulty.

On taking up post both politicians and Chief Executive were clear that change was required of a magnitude that the council was singularly ill prepared for – both in terms of culture and available resource. For Henshaw the transformational potential of harnessing new technologies in order to create a new Liverpool dynamic was clearly a key strategic plank in his reform agenda. However, an external review commissioned in 2000 revealed the chronic lack of investment in infrastructure projects that had occurred in the previous decade. A recommendation was made that the council consider entering in to an outsourcing relationship with a service provider; a model already adopted by a number of local government organisations in the United Kingdom, and indeed an approach not uncommon in many other countries. Taking this 'solution'-focused route may well have been the obvious path for an organisation struggling to move itself to a more stable operating position, yet Henshaw's immediate instinct appears to have been to consider a culture where bolder and essentially more entrepreneurial thinking was encouraged; as one senior manager commented, 'he didn't want to outsource the problems, his view was that we should insource the solution'. A critical review of other outsourcing projects within the local government context had left in Henshaw some sense that, as traditionally configured, they led both constituents in the partnership primarily focused upon matters of contract rather than the underpinning aims and goals.

The approach advocated by Henshaw to move the council forward in its aims to re-engineer services through harnessing all appropriate technological channels was to adapt the joint venture approach, which is often deployed in large-scale commercial sector activities. Liverpool Direct Limited (LDL) was thus formed, after a lengthy period of discussion with a number of interested parties, with the UK telecoms giant, BT, as the strategic partner. Configured under local government's strict financial guidelines, LDL is a joint venture company, owned 80 per cent by BT and 20 per cent by the council. For BT the attractions of entering into such a novel arrangement were clearly around building a reputation in a market segment which they saw as being potentially attractive to them over the medium and longer term, as well as having the opportunity to interact with a public service at a more strategic level than would normally be the case in an outsourcing relationship. Critically LDL offered BT the opportunity to learn more about the realities of public services working, cultures and behaviours; factors which they felt would help them to position themselves strongly in an expanding market.

Now some three years old, the LDL model remains largely a novelty in local government terms in the UK – although much visited, there appears to be some nervousness even today around entering into such an innovative and risk-sharing environment, although others are actively engaged in seeking some variance to this approach. However, analysis of the terms of the joint venture proposition would tend to suggest that the relationship entered into has been based upon mutual confidence with the commercial partner holding, it would appear, a far greater proportion of the associated risks. The concept of genuine partnership is enhanced still further by the fact that the LDL's Chief Executive also holds an executive portfolio within the council – his joint citizenship, like those of the staff who work under the LDL umbrella, is guaranteed. Such an approach to staffing, guaranteeing all staff working within LDL services the rights to return to council employment should they choose to do so, was extremely helpful in setting a collaborative and non-confrontational agenda both with employees and their unions.

Configured on a ten-year contractual model the underpinning requirements of LDL's business model are that all information and communications technology requirements are covered; as are the start-up and running costs of a customer contact centre; human resources and payroll and benefits services. In return for this BT are guaranteed an annual payment of some £30 million over the ten-year period of the agreement. Their strategy in responding to the challenges of this ambitious agenda has been to acknowledge the need to front-load their investment in the council and its infrastructure. This has involved not only large-scale investment in technological platforms for change but also significant investments in business process re-engineering reviews and major cultural change programmes. Their calculated risk has been that by adopting this early investment push, which they argue has so far cost them more per annum than they receive from the council, they will accrue significant cost reductions in the second half of the contracted time period, such that they will move comfortably into profit within the LDL framework.

By 2003 the improvements gained through approaches and invest-ment made over only a two-year period appear commendable. Even allowing for a degree of commercial hyperbole it is important to note key service gains:

'Improved revenue collection has been achieved with record levels of council tax and business rates collected . . .

The service's overarching performance management framework has ensured that increased focus is placed on LDL's top asset, its people. Each member of staff receives regular feedback and opportunities to develop in their role. Skill levels have been improved as the new ICT systems have been implemented with the support of comprehensive training programmes . . .

LDL is investing over £5 million in systems for Business Rates, Council Tax and Housing Benefit. These new systems cover core applications used to produce bills and make payments and new systems that support the business with electronic case management and workflow. This has enabled us to transform our ability to resolve customer enquiries at the first point of contact with up to minute access to the latest customer documentation . . .

The Resourcing Team is responsible for the co-ordination of the recruitment process from vacancy referral through to appointment. This also involves the management of the temporary staff "Pool" and the processing of Criminal Records Bureau checks. The team manages the re-deployment process . . .. This process has been particularly successful accruing savings of some £21 million over the last three years . . .'

(Liverpool Direct Ltd 2003)

That can point to all of these activities as being key to the aspirations of Henshaw and the wider city council membership, to radically transform the organisational 'architecture', in such a way that new ways of working which are citizen- and partner-focused become the 'norm'. However, as other transformation-focused local government organisations have found internationally, a key plank in achieving a changed external perception is through radical refocusing of those areas of activity which see greatest engagement with citizens. To this end, it is no surprise that a key focus of the LDL proposition has been upon achieving radical change to the customer contact channels previously offered. As has been the case in other beacon sites of local government change, such as Brisbane City Council in Australia, a key driver for change was the move to integrate call centre approaches into the service design (Milner 2002: 63–85).

'In just four years, Liverpool Direct has evolved from a traditional local authority switchboard passing incoming calls straight through to back office services, to a 300-seater customer service hub handling over 180,000 calls a month . . .

The contact centre is a key element of LDL. The centre provides total access to the citizens of Liverpool giving them an extensive range of services provided by the Council. It is the first point of contact and aims to offer the resolution to all enquiries from members of the public. Their aim is front-end call resolution, so that every call is satisfied at the first point of contact and the customer does not have to call back. Currently they resolve 86% of calls at the first point of contact. The centre also aims to answer 90% of calls within 20 seconds and consistently exceeds this target.

Residents access the contact centre by phone, fax or email, through one-stop shops in the City – from 2002 it moved to offer contact 24 × 7 × 365.

The contact centre is based on teams of around 17 full and part-time workers. Work is team focused. Trust and empowerment are key aspects of working as a team. Each team is led by a team coach, who reports to an operations manager. The centre places strong emphasis on training and development . . .

The contact centre also has a career progression scheme that rewards high achievers, encouraging them to speed up their progression through the salary bands . . .

In addition to handling general enquiries, ranging from obtaining a disabled car parking permit to finding a local councillor, the contact centre seeks to resolve a wide range of enquiries ranging from the street scene (cleaning, lighting, abandoned vehicles) through registrar services and benefits . . .. New services are continually added on to the contact centres brief. There is a dedicated team, the Business Transformation Team, whose role is to bring in new services, design and adapt the re-engineered procedures for delivery and consistently review and redesign them.'

(Liverpool Direct Ltd 2003)

As was the case with the Brisbane model of local government reform, a key aspiration, having established a robust internal architecture for information flow and exchange, was to look externally for opportunities for undertaking work on behalf of partner organisations. A key aspiration for Liverpool was not only should they cover the costs of partnership working, indeed returning a satisfactory operating profit remains a clear goal, but that they should be able to demonstrate the benefits to citizens accruing from being able to facilitate system-wide delivery of public services. Examples of such partnership working include close liaison with the local police force around the management of abandoned vehicles:

'Abandoned vehicles are a blot on inner city landscapes causing environmental and public safety concerns. It engenders an image of deprivation and poverty. The swift removal of such vehicles minimises associated crime and demonstrates to residents that the City Council is a responsible authority. By providing a contact point through Liverpool Direct reports are expedited quickly, relieve the emergency services of non-emergency calls, and assist in the prompt removal of the vehicle. It is acknowledged that the estimated cost to a local authority of dealing with damage etc., associated with abandoned vehicles could be as high as £11,000 per vehicle. This cost includes any repairs to highways due to fires, damage etc. The potential annual cost to the Authority runs into hundreds of thousands of pounds. The prompt removal of abandoned vehicles (within 48 hours) now results in significant road repair budget savings. Merseyside Police have also acknowledged that the initiative has had a 25% reduction in vehicle related crime within the city.'

(Liverpool City Council 2003)

Abandoned cars represent only one small part of the network of wider public and voluntary service working that the LDL systems architecture and capability has made possible. However, what such an example signals is that this model of working has been a major catalyst for breaking away from traditional and rather limiting ways of working, which has often resulted with various 'arms' of public service provision giving the appearance of being somewhat disjointed. Demonstrating the strategic and operational capacity to look beyond the confines of their own direct service remit, Liverpool City Council has shown itself to be a highly innovative instigator of service transformation. However, even in what may be termed these relatively early days, it is important to identify that although there have been some tremendous advances associated with LDL, there are, in respect particularly of considering the capacity of the council to move beyond a change agenda and into the realms of renewal, some concerns which demand consideration.

Clearly, as we have said, in its relatively short life-span LDL has been a hugely successful catalyst for change within the Liverpool City Council service brief. As a business model it reflects the innovative and 'can do' attitude of the Chief Executive, and has served to create a sense of real improvement and achievement around the council which, as we discussed earlier in this chapter, is far removed from the image of an organisation that was only 20 years ago a beacon for advocates of extremism and political excess. Yet, it is possible to argue that as the change agenda matures, and the move towards embedding the potential for renewal becomes a real possibility, the LDL as a service-providing structure could be seen as problematic.

Renewal, as we discussed in Chapters 3 and 4, is reliant upon embedding new cultures, beliefs and behaviours *across* an organisation. For public sector organisations this is particularly challenging, as they are usually complex and often underpinned by an ethos which whilst not necessarily automatically resistant to change, is often profoundly suspicious of it. The LDL model represents a response to an immediate problem arising from service neglect; in as much as it has addressed and remedied key service priorities, it has clearly been successful. Yet, one must remember that LDL is *not* Liverpool City Council; certainly, it enacts key services on its behalf, but residing within the council remain such services as Education and Social Services, where the vast majority of employees remain employed. Leading change and renewal in areas such as these, which do not lend themselves easily to improvement-focused metrics, is in reality where the key leadership challenges remain in Liverpool. Whilst celebrating the success of LDL, one is left wondering what the impact has been upon those services not operating under its umbrella.

An interesting perspective upon the LDL and other services dichotomy was provided by having the opportunity to question staff from both constituencies. Interestingly both were in complete agreement that a key issue that they felt was impinging upon the council's ability to move forward, was the marked difference in cultures that were felt to exist across the two operating structures. LDL's emergent culture was cited as being increasingly different to that of the rest of the council; with its high emphasis upon prioritising personal development and responsibility for service delivery at a relatively junior level, it was held up to be everything that the rest of the council was not. LDL was cited as being focused upon publicly recognising and thanking staff for their contribution to change and success, yet we were told that for services outside LDL, 'saying thank you is not something Liverpool City Council does'. Such a statement whilst in itself a powerful criticism of a two-tier culture that appears to have evolved since the creation of LDL, does also raise some important questions around where leadership and intervention are actually occurring. Recalling not only that LDL is a joint venture company in which the council is a significant stakeholder, but also that the Chief Executive of LDL is also an executive portfolio holder within the main council body, one wonders why such key cultural challenges have not been highlighted and acted upon to a greater extent. This would appear particularly ironic given that the Audit Commission's assessment of the council drew particular attention to its ability to evidence a capacity to *learn*.

The LDL approach has done much to move Liverpool City Council forward from a basis of failure to one of performance and service enhancement. To some extent it is possible to argue, as critics both internal and external have done, that this was a project that neither the council nor the commercial sector partner could allow to fail. For both, the premiums accruing from successful outcomes were significant, in terms of reputation and credibility, so latitude has perhaps been deployed over contractual exactitude when it has been necessary to do so. Again, this would seem perfectly appropriate given the particular circumstances into which LDL was launched. However, that it could potentially serve to destabilise the council's ability to innovate and drive forward service enhancement at the 'harder' end of the public service food chain, is undoubtedly a very real risk. This risk should be characterised as accruing from the sense that parallel cultures have grown up in a relatively short time, with the LDL culture, focused on a high regard for the individual, standing in some degree of contrast to the more traditional collective responsibility for silo-based services that appears extant across the rest of the council.

David Henshaw's view of the future of public service provision appears to be based upon a belief that there are certain circumstances in which it is appropriate to 'pass the baton' by which is meant demonstrating an awareness that simply because an organisation has a history of delivering a service, is no longer a justification for this always being so. With all the risks around parallel cultures that have been raised here, it is also important to acknowledge that the degree of change required in an organisation such as Liverpool City Council, would, whatever the approach deployed, have problems associated with it. The greatest risk, taking a longitudinal perspective, would have been in 1999 to make a conscious decision to do nothing. The emergence of partnership working and of a more genuinely mixed economy in the provision of public services, demonstrates that, whatever the current limitations and concerns, the LDL approach is one that has delivered net gains for Liverpool in terms of the quality of services delivered to its citizens.

THE LIVERPOOL WAY – DEVELOPING LEADERSHIP CAPABILITY

If LDL represents one strand of the Liverpool change and renewal process then certainly the approach referred to internally as 'the Liverpool Way' represents, at the very least, an attempt to balance the service reform agenda with a focus on the capabilities and competencies of the employees. Interestingly, having reflected upon the key issue of parallel cultures that emerged from scrutiny of the LDL approach, it is worth noting the council's own description of its investment in people and their development:

> 'We have made great strides in ensuring our staff feel valued and are developed as this has a major influence on how they interact with customers. To do this we have invested heavily in staff training and development. We have responded to staff surveys by introducing a three-year development programme called "The Liverpool Way" which has been designed to build a much more effective workplace and introduce new ways to work together and communicate with each other. If the city council is to improve its services, meet higher levels of customer satisfaction and quality, and achieve its vision of "putting the customer at the heart of everything we do" then we have to change old habits and mindsets. We have to create a new culture through changing the way we work. The "Liverpool Way" is the city council's public demonstration of our commitment to help the organisation achieve real improvement in service delivery, customer satisfaction and quality. It is focussed on encouraging greater integrity and transparency and on building respect and trust. Every employee participates in the programme.'
>
> (Liverpool City Council 2003)

Aside from his obvious commitment to investing in the Liverpool City Council workforce, Henshaw is acknowledged as being a skilful and persuasive communicator. Many of those who participated in this study referred to his inspirational and charismatic leadership style, which they felt was evidenced through his performance at staff roadshows, regular emails to all colleagues and the general tone that he set as Chief Executive. Interestingly, in reflecting back to the beginning of Henshaw's career as CEO, it was honesty in the face of adversity which appeared to have been a key early indicator to colleagues that this was someone who actually meant to 'do business'. From the outset he was held to have been honest and 'upfront', reportedly telling an early meeting of senior and middle management colleagues, 'Half of you won't be here next year.' Whilst this can appear on the surface to be rather a harsh statement, it was held by those who had been party to it, to have been helpful in building a sense that here was someone who might not have all the answers but who was determined to address the issues which had built over the past decades of neglect.

In essence the Liverpool Way appears to be a formalised mechanism for ensuring two key priorities: one being that the council is equipped with a staffing base which is both competent and capable of taking forward the ongoing change agenda. The second is rather more subtle, but relates to building and engendering a capacity for *following* within the workforce. The latter point is in danger of slipping into Machiavellian interpretation and requires careful clarification of what the concept of followership actually involves within an evolving context such as this. Taking note of terms used to describe Henshaw's style which have included 'directive', 'charismatic' and 'inspirational' we have a clear sense that here is an organisation that can be said to have a highly credible leader and an apparently well-respected executive team around him. However, there is potentially an argument which suggests that direction, charisma and reflection can take an organisation only so far – and that possibly this is the stage that Liverpool had reached by 2003.

The Liverpool Way project can be characterised as a response to a maturing organisational scenario. Profound change based around organisational reshaping has been largely achieved, things both look and feel different. Moving into a period of sustained renewal, however, is likely to require that new behaviours and beliefs become embedded across the organisation and this requires greater consideration than is often found in public service organisations. Henshaw's decision to send a major signal around the value of the council staff to the future shape and success of the organisation, through the decision to invest in the workforce, is far more powerful than relying upon vision or values statements, albeit that in some instances they result in laminated cards which are dutifully filed and then largely forgotten. If we reflect upon the organisational renewal theory introduced in Chapter 4 we can see that having a formalised focus upon the employee represents a substantial investment in attempting to inculcate the vision and values of a continuously evolving organisation over an extended period of time.

Deciding to invest in the development of confident, competent and committed employees represents a second plank in the change and renewal journey of Liverpool City Council. Although too recent a decision to evaluate against any meaningful metrics, the decision in itself is an important signal as to the direction of travel. The creation of LDL opened up opportunities for Liverpool to actually do things differently and to be able to demonstrate the benefits of doing so. However, as we discussed, there have been some significant concerns emerging around the impact of this business model upon the large majority of staff and service areas which do not fall directly under the re-engineering focus of LDL. Investing in *all* staff and opening up a development stream which prioritises building a capacity for continuous innovation, problem-solving and cross-boundary working is one way of ensuring that the next phase of Liverpool life-cycle is based upon locking in key staff con-stituencies to a culture and aspirational mind-set that delineates them as followers of a new type of public service ethos. The focus upon *follower-ship* that is being built through this process is arguably not one of slavish adherence to rigid sets of beliefs or principles; but rather it should be characterised by a willingness to acknowledge the paramount impor-tance of the public service mission, whilst having the flexibility and willingness to embrace many and varied models of actual delivery.

AMBITION IS GOOD – LIVERPOOL EUROPEAN CAPITAL OF CULTURE

At the outset of this chapter we shared the thought put forward by a city council manager that the progress made by Liverpool as a local government organisation, was amply reflected by the amount of national recognition it was now gaining for innovative and improvement-focused practice. Indeed when quantified the scale of recognition achieved is impressive:

> 'Over the last two years we have been visited by over 213 Local Authorities, Central Government departments and private companies to see how we have managed our phenomenal transition. We are continually sharing examples of good practice with our colleagues in other authorities to help improve customer service nationwide.'
>
> (Liverpool City Council 2003)

However, the ambition of Liverpool to demonstrate its ability to be a place to 'do business' has moved beyond the national agenda and into the spheres of international recognition. When the opportunity arose early in Henshaw's tenure as Chief Executive for cities in England to bid for the status of European City of Culture in 2008, he was clear in his view that Liverpool should bid for this title, and indeed not only bid, but do so with the expectation of succeeding. In terms of context, the City of Culture programme is run through the European Union, with member states taking turns to nominate a city for designation in an agreed year. In terms of profile-raising and oppor-tunities for regeneration, Henshaw had only to look to the impact that being designated a city of culture had had upon cities such as Glasgow and Dublin, to realise that this was something that he and key political colleagues wanted for Liverpool.

Competition for this award is typically very strong and in terms of those English cities bidding for the 2008 award, certainly taken very seriously. The bids, which were received and assessed by the

Department for Culture, Media and Sport, came from other major centres of population such as Birmingham. Liverpool's bid proposition was based upon highlighting its long history as a culturally diverse centre of trade; its prowess and pride in its sporting history and its established links to key developments in music and the arts. However, what set the bid apart from its competitors was arguably the focus upon pride and passion in the city, both in its past and in a vision of where it wanted to be. Had Liverpool not been awarded the designation of capital of culture there would certainly have been high levels of disappointment; however, as one local politician commented:

> 'Just bidding was a Liverpool success story, the fact that we were able to put in what most agreed was a courageous and serious bid was a sign of growing confidence and ambition; being awarded capital of culture status represents a real maturing of the change agenda. For somewhere that only a few years ago was typically held to be the benchmark for poverty of ambition this really has been a miracle.'

It is interesting to note the number of occasions the term 'miracle' is used when considering Liverpool City Council through the eyes of both internal and external stakeholders. The term in itself denotes something unexpected, possibly held to be outside the realms of reasonable possibility and, when one considers Liverpool's starting-point, it is perhaps indicative of the journey that Henshaw commenced only 4 years ago. The capital of culture bid was nothing short of an act of faith, underpinned largely by a glorious but not necessarily fully developed or enabled vision of a city that could take on such large-scale challenges. Winning the bid has meant a further stage in building organisational confidence has been gained – Liverpool City Council has been entrusted with steering a role which is internationally focused.

LIVERPOOL RENEWAL OR SHORT-LIVED MIRACLE?

In terms of the capacity for moving towards attaining the ability for the organisation to continually renew itself, the capital of culture award, taken together with the other change activities outlined so far within this chapter, represent what Tushman refers to as the 'transition period' (Tushman and O'Reilly 2002: 184). What this term points us towards is the existence of a renewal-orientated trajectory which sees the management of change and the cultural impacts associated with this, as being one stage in a journey that sees an organisation developing the capacity to renew and reshape emerging over time. In the case of Liverpool the transition phase appears to have been well thought through, although it is possible to argue that, at least in part, the planning has been less important that the actual execution and communication. By this what is meant is that the transition phase bears the hallmarks of personal vision and leadership as being key inputs. Tushman argues that the success or otherwise of this phase of the renewal journey has much to do with both speed and leadership:

> 'The transition period is particularly crucial . . .. During the transition, managers and their teams take the organization apart and, component by component, move it toward the future. Given the politics, individual resistance to change, and control issues during transition periods, the shorter the period the better . . .. A poorly managed transition process puts future organizational performance at risk.'
>
> (Tushman and O'Reilly 2002: 184)

Henshaw's approach to the transition phase has certainly involved unpicking organisational structures and cultures. It has also been, given the scale of reshaping involved, in public service terms, an impressively fast change process. Gaining investment in infrastructure and people, improving key stakeholder relationships and going after a major external project have been key building blocks in building an organisation which is both competent and confident. Yet, a key question remains around the capacity to renew, to keep working towards revised views of the future, and that is simply what would happen if David Henshaw was taken out of the Liverpool equation? Recalling that the concept of renewal is founded upon organisational maturity at almost every level, one has to ask whether, after some four years in post, Liverpool can move beyond a point where a frequently articulated view within the organisation is that 'David Henshaw is Liverpool City Council'. Whilst not wishing to build a sense of a personality cult across the organisation, a clear message emerging from interviews held across the council, was that for many the motivation for and direction of travel around change and change processes, appeared reliant upon having a clear articulation from the very top. Such a reliance upon strong leadership is entirely understandable given that the starting-point for the transition process was one of profound organisational fragility. Linking back once more to the quasi-religious terminology of the 'miraculous' journey, it is important to acknowledge the type and style of visionary leadership that Henshaw has deployed so successfully.

In terms of Henshaw's leadership contribution, it is significant to note that the most important characteristic that he exemplified at the outset of his relationship with Liverpool City Council was the fact that he was a *leader*. In an environment that had been riven by political extremism, to have a leadership figure who was actually interested in the organisation, its mission and responsibility to all stakeholders, was demonstrably different. To have one who exuded passion for, and belief in, a public service ethos which was service- and customer-driven rather than politically framed, was again something quite unique in the Liverpool experience. The picture painted of Henshaw is therefore almost messianic in terms of his personal impact, and this is a view that is not unreasonable within the transition phase of a renewal model, where the role of visionary leaders is often held to be critical:

'Visionary leaders are able to mobilize and sustain energy and activity within an organization by taking specific personal actions. Visionary leaders are not popular versions of the great speech makers or television personalities. Visionary leadership is not equivalent to charisma. Rather, visionary leaders are able to emotionally engage their organization at whatever level they operate. . . . Visionary leaders energize the organization and find ways to motivate its members to achieve its goals. They demonstrate empathy, listen, understand and share the feelings of others in the organization. They express their confidence in their own ability and the ability of others to succeed. They create events to signal and celebrate transitions and turning points, expressing support for individuals grappling with the pressures of stressful change efforts and reinforcing the new vision and culture.

The behaviours associated with visionary leadership support innovation and change in several ways. Visionary leaders provide a psychological focal point for the energies, hopes and aspirations of people in the organization. They serve as powerful role models whose actions and personal energy demonstrate the desired behaviours. Their behaviour is a standard to which others can aspire. Through their commitment, effectiveness and consistency, visionary leaders build a personal bond between themselves and the organization.'
(Tushman and O'Reilly 2002: 185–6)

Against all of these descriptors of leadership David Henshaw is a truly high performer. Perhaps most striking is the concept of a 'personal bond' being built between the leader and the organisation. Here there is certainly clear resonance with the views expressed by his colleagues that Henshaw the leader, and Liverpool City Council, the organisational entity, are one and the same. For the successful roll-out of a transition phase such an emphasis upon visionary leadership has undoubtedly been a key, if not in fact *the* key, component of the change journey. So far so good then, the journey towards renewal appears to be ongoing. However, questions do remain, and these are largely around the extent to which the organisation is developing capacity to change and renew organically. Can in fact Henshaw demonstrate the ability to be an adaptive leader as well as a visionary one?

In terms of the time-frames of this case study, it is simply too early to tell whether Liverpool will be capable of following a renewal path, or whether like many other organisations that have gone through successful phases of change, it will at some point elect to pursue a stability strategy. The dangers of the latter, whilst undoubtedly appealing to many who have had to work with almost continuous change processes and challenges, is that stability is illusory, and that even a *pause* can result in having to commence the change and transition phase once again. From analysis of the Liverpool journey to date, it seems unlikely that Henshaw is instinctively drawn to stability. However, what is perhaps more difficult to judge is the extent to which he is personally capable of making adjustments to his own leadership style such that there is possibly greater emphasis upon managing the short-term change imperatives through focusing upon developing longer-term organisational competencies. Evidence of such adaptation might usefully be a greater organisational awareness of a senior team, rather than a single leader which was certainly a perception that was voiced by a majority of participants making input to this review.

Thus, research benefiting from greater opportunities for longitudinal analysis than this, will be helpful in gauging the success or otherwise of the Liverpool City Council journey. However, as a case study in leadership it is important in terms of the learning opportunities it provides. Taking an organisation which was the subject of widespread vilification and transforming it to the point where it has demonstrably improved, to an extent whereby aspects of service are held to be beacon sites of innovation and good practice, is a success story measured against almost every management metric. To create an environment where the scope, scale and pace of change enacted has been once again at an extreme end of any organisational 'wish list' is once again hugely laudable. And yet, for the longer term, questions remain, just as they do for all successful and innovative organisations regardless of their sector. How to sustain this sense of moving forward without falling into the dangers of innovation fatigue or exhaustion of organisational capacity to deal with complex change issues?

The key concepts advocated in earlier chapters of this work, those of renewal and adaptation, are important considerations to deploy when looking ahead to the next stage of Liverpool's development. The transition from failing organisation to innovative and generally successful public service-focused entity appears to have been successfully negotiated. That process has been driven by visionary leadership which both internally and externally has been commented upon for its highly directional nature. New ways of working, such as the creation of LDL, the investment that the Liverpool Way development and communication strategy represents, arguably suggest an organisation that is planning for a less directional approach to the future. However, what no amount of future gazing can account for, is the extent to which David Henshaw as an obviously successful leader, is both capable and willing to adapt his own style with a view to allowing greater local leadership to evidence itself across the organisation. Whatever the future holds, the one certainty is that the achievements of 1999–2004 in leadership and change terms place Liverpool amongst all too small a group of organisations that have managed to achieve organisational transformation.

VOICES ON LEADERSHIP – 'COMMENTS BY DAVID HENSHAW'

As part of the case study process, David Henshaw was invited to contribute his views on the key leadership challenges facing public services. What follows is an input from a highly respected 'voice' on leadership.

Britain's public services face unprecedented challenges at the start of the 21st century. Leaders are being asked to deliver more modern, efficient and dynamic services at a time of great social and technological change. And public sector leaders face external constraints that are different from those of the private sector.

People want public services which meet their needs, when they need it. People are exercising choice and demanding higher quality. In the private sector, service standards and service delivery have improved as a result. People are now rightly demanding a better service not just from the private sector, but from the public sector too.

We need to be able to respond to the expectations of our citizens and adapt to the needs of users. Innovation is the key to improving performance in public services and increasing public value. Information technology is revolutionising our lives, including the way we work, the way we communicate and the way we learn. New technologies offer opportunities to engage with customers in new ways and redesign back offices to improve efficient delivery; increasing service efficiency whilst minimising costs.

What does it take to achieve organisational turnaround so that public services are truly customer-focused? We must unleash the potential within the public service to drive our modernising agenda forward. We need a clear understanding of what behaviours work in delivering today's public services. Clear accountability for performance needs to be matched by greater freedom to lead. But strong leadership also involves real commitment from all partners. The leadership of partnerships is not just about building connections between the various stakeholders, it is about baton changing and being clear about exactly what you are trying to achieve.

We need a vision for success that is harnessing new technology to facilitate change and lead local governance; delivering public services to meet the needs of citizens, not the convenience of the service providers.

CHAPTER 8

LESSONS IN LEADERSHIP

INTRODUCTION

In this final chapter on leadership in the public services we want to draw out three things that have been addressed in this book. These are the problem leadership is meant to solve, the processes through which leadership is enacted, and the relationship between managers and elected politicians in the course of leadership. Then we set out nine lessons in leadership.

THE PROBLEM LEADERSHIP ADDRESSES

In our opinion, the main problem leadership in the public services is addressing is the remaking of the social-democratic welfare state society into a new welfare state society, and the key role of leaders is adapting the public services in that transition. To understand this problem better we can take a look at the origins and history of the welfare state modern societies. We will do this by taking Britain as our example.

The early 1930s were an economic disaster for Britain and many other countries, but this was against a backdrop of persistently high unemployment in the inter-war years. Beveridge's book *Full Employment in a Free Society* (1944) reported a general unemployment rate in Great Britain and Northern Ireland in 1931 and 1932 of over 20 per cent but between 1921 and 1938 it averaged 14.2 per cent. One result was poverty. Large numbers of families had the bare minimum for existence or less. G. D. H. Cole summed up the situation as follows:

'There were at all times literally millions looking for jobs and unable to find them; and in face of the plain fact of poverty, implying the need for all that could be produced, the whole capitalist world was persistently wasting productive resources and letting men and women rot away in idleness instead of setting them to useful work.'

(Cole 1947: 324)

The Beveridge Report of 1942, described by Cole as one of the great social documents of the day, contained proposals for giving security of income in the face of an event or situation that spelt the end of income from earning. Unemployment, disability, retirement, maternity, and widowhood were all envisaged as relevant claims for financial support. Each locality in Britain was to get a Security Office to provide cash benefits to process claims. The payment of benefit was to continue for as long as the need existed. The security offered through this scheme was to be for every one of Britain's citizens – rich and poor. Everyone was to contribute directly an equal amount to fund this social insurance. However, the rich would then pay through tax since the state also contributed a share of the funding. Beveridge also proposed benefits to be paid based on the number of children in the family (children's allowances) and he made the establishment of a Public Health Service for the whole population an assumption of his social insurance proposals. Beveridge (1944: 17) summed up his intentions in his 1942 report as follows:

> 'The Plan for Social Security is designed to secure . . . that every individual . . . shall have an income sufficient for the healthy subsistence of himself and his family, an income to keep him above Want, when for any reason he cannot work and earn . . . the Report proposes children's allowances to ensure that, however large the family, no child shall ever be in Want, and medical treatment of all kinds for all persons when sick, without a charge on treatment, to ensure that no person need be sick because he has not the means to pay the doctor or the hospital.'

In his 1944 book Beveridge outlined a policy for full employment (which he defined as not more than 3 per cent unemployed) and suggested that the war had demonstrated the benefits of the 'socialization of demand without socialization of production' (1944: 17). He proposed dealing with the problem of unemployment in peace time by making the state responsible for the sufficiency of demand in the economy, which he saw as including being concerned with both public and private investment.

At the time, Beveridge's proposals on social insurance, public health services, and his policy for maintaining full employment must have seemed to many working class people and communities like Utopia, having lived through the misery of mass unemployment and poverty in the 1930s. It represented a package of proposals that outlined how the state could deliver to them security and support from all the key uncertainties and risks of life. The report at the time it was submitted to government was expected to entail increased spending by government and costs for employers. Progress would have its price. The social insurance scheme implied rises in public spending, including on pensions. It implied increased labour costs for employers, although Beveridge thought that higher costs in this case would be more than covered by increased efficiency and work that employers would get in return. The report had critics. Cole claimed that:

> 'there were not wanting critics on the Tory side who asserted that Great Britain could not afford it. These same critics in many cases also disliked the plan, because they thought that it involved too much state help to the poor and the workers, and might "undermine the incentives to labour" or unduly strengthen the hands of the Trade Unions in wage-bargaining, or, more generally, mollycoddle the people, who ought to maintain themselves by their own efforts.'
>
> (Cole 1947: 545)

For the most part, according to Cole, the critics did not come out into the open. The Labour Government passed legislation on social security and legislation on a National Health Service in 1946, creating the basis of the post-war welfare state, and, until the 1970s, Britain went on to enjoy full employment. Utopia had been achieved. Or had it?

The spending on the welfare state could be an economic burden on 'society' or it could be economically functional. As an example of the second view, Beveridge thought the spending on the health service was an investment and would pay for itself because people would become fitter and Britain would be more productive. So while it might normally be assumed that employing people in the public services is a financial cost society bears on the basis of the wealth-creating sector of the economy, such an expenditure can be an investment if the effect is to raise private sector productivity.

After many years of the proportion of the population covered by income tax steadily rising, the welfare state became more controversial. More and more people questioned whether Britain could afford to spend so much on welfare. In the 1990s the welfare state was poised in a difficult position. On one hand it was seen as a financial burden and many people were concerned about media stories of scroungers on welfare. On the other hand, cutting back on welfare and reducing the National Health Service was politically unacceptable. The position was a stalemate. Hence the move to a new welfare state society is an attempt to find a temporary resolution of the economic and political tensions. The nature of the new welfare state is not completely clear, but from the case studies in this book we might suggest that it is based on several propositions. First, the welfare state is needed because individuals at various stages in their life may need support, for example if they become unemployed. Second, the support needs to be provided in a way that does not foster dependence but independence. Third, the welfare state needs to provide services for the many and not the few. We saw in the case of Newham Council that the many may include the needy but it also includes more affluent groups as well. Fourth, the changes in the welfare state necessitate reconstructing the relationship of the public services to the public so that the public experience their services as treating them with dignity and taking their needs and problems seriously. The dignity of the experience was one of the issues in the Jobcentre Plus case study. If recent history suggests the reconstruction of the relationship cannot be done through representative democracy alone, then the new welfare state society will experiment with using public consultation and offering service users choice as a way of making the relationship a better one. Fifth, serving the public better implies challenges to the status quo within public services organisations, and working through the problems that existing cultures are posing, in order to develop radical solutions. This might mean confronting resistance such as that at Middlesbrough Council or in Jobcentre Plus, or bringing into being new services such as those pioneered in Centrelink. If all these propositions can be made to come true, then the public services in a modern democracy will become a means by which the individual is made stronger using the support of society. There is in other words no necessary antagonism between individualism and collectivism. Some of the findings of the Jobcentre Plus case study indicate that there has been a conscious political project to reconstruct the welfare state society in Britain using this new model.

But the culture and structures, and the resistance of professionals within the welfare state, do make moving to the new welfare state a challenge. There is a problem of resistance to the loss of some features of the old welfare state. So we conclude that it is important to go beyond the idea that leadership in the public services is just about change (which is what everyone says). This change is a specific one. It is about reforms that bring a new accommodation between social democracy and the economy in the 21st century. Because of the scale of the changes required it requires high-quality managerial leadership, and widespread confidence in it. We are guessing that in far too many public services organisations today we would find employees who felt that changes had not been explained to them and that they had not been given any opportunity to express their views or give feedback on the changes. We would no doubt also find many where employees felt unprepared for the changes and felt that no one was concerned about the consequences of change for them. However inaccurate these feelings might be, their effects would be no less real.

LEADERSHIP PROCESSES

The leadership processes that are currently dominant in the public services appear to be aimed at adapting and modernising a welfare state society. This means paying attention to productivity as well as making step changes in the nature of the services and reconstructing the relationship with the public. The constituent processes are not just summed up by vision, inspiration and empowerment (which is a common account of visionary leadership). But in practice, it also needs thorough knowledge of the business of the public service, skills in stakeholder management and conflict management, a willingness to confront the difficulty of taking managers and employees out of their comfort zones, and detailed planning and detailed checking on the execution of the plans. We would also make a distinction between visionary leaders that have a morally uplifting effect on their followers and leaders who create trust by demonstrating genuine concern for the people they lead.

Table 8.1 Visionary and Adaptive Leadership.

Visionary	and	Thoroughly grounded knowledge of the business
Inspiring	and	Skilled in stakeholder management/conflict management/taking people out of their comfort zones
Empowering	and	Detailed planning and rigorous monitoring of actions and performance
Morally uplifting	and	Genuine concern for the people they lead

MANAGERS AND ELECTED POLITICIANS

Lesson One: managerial leaders adapt to political leadership

We now draw out leadership lessons in respect of the relationship between managers and politicians. We single this relationship out for attention because it is what is specific to leadership in the public services as against leadership in the private sector. The table (Table 8.2) implies some different relationships between elected politicians and the managerial leaders. This is drawn directly from the case studies analysed in Chapter 6 and uses an earlier conceptualisation of leadership action in a period of strategic change (Joyce 2000: 15).

The first case study in Chapter 6 concerned Middlesbrough Council. The organisation was in no state to be innovative – it was in a financial crisis. A new Chief Executive was headhunted to bring about change but initially he chose to 'take responsibility' for solving the financial crisis. It shows that in some circumstances elected politicians need managerial leaders who can sort out problems thereby making it possible for organisations to be receptive to change. The second case was different. The council was in a sense ready for change. The councillors wanted to be aligned with the new government's reform agenda. They had some ideas but had not yet crystallised them into a strategic vision. They hired a new Chief Executive who was able to create a strategic vision, which the councillors voted to adopt. This was not the Chief Executive's vision so much as a vision that 'completed' their ideas. This case shows that in some circumstances elected politicians need managerial leaders who can take the politicians' political aspirations and turn them into visions and strategies. The final case showed that there is yet a third possibility. This is when elected politicians need managerial leaders who will provide visible leadership and carry through to a conclusion the changes they have envisioned. The new Chief Executive came in and 'fronted' vision and also developed its detail in a way that would help staff to buy into it.

Table 8.2 Processual View of Public Services Leadership.

STAGE IN CHANGE PROCESS	WHAT CHIEF EXECUTIVE DID
PREPARING FOR CHANGE Creating a situation in which organisation can be receptive to change	Took 'responsibility' for solving financial crisis
LEADING CHANGE Creating goals/vision and involving others and installing management	Prepared vision statement that political leadership wanted – 'completed' their thinking
CHANGING Aligning the organisation with the strategic vision, changing budgets and activities etc. – bringing people along with the vision	'Fronted' the politicians' vision – was visible leader in period of implementation

Using the three case studies it is clear that effective leadership is based on strong political support for the managerial leadership at the top of the organisation. But the specifics of the relationship between the managerial leader and the political leadership could be seen as one in which the managerial leadership adapts itself to the political leadership and in a sense complements it. This is the first lesson respecting the relationship between managers and elected politicians: effective managerial leaders adapt to and complement political leadership.

Lesson Two: leaders manage conflict

Managerial leaders may find changing the culture involves them in managing conflict that has its origins in the democratic process and its mediation of the interests of those who produce the public services and those who use the public services. The Middlesbrough case study illustrated that very well. The council had taken on managers and staff in the context of a commitment to no compulsory redundancy. But this implied a financial burden that was leading to a crisis. If the public were not prepared to fund this commitment, there was no option but to make people redundant. Why should people in Middlesbrough be prepared to do this? Unemployment was a problem in the area and the citizens in general had not been guaranteed employment, so why should they morally feel obliged to underwrite complete security for those they employed to provide services collectively to the community? The series of well-attended public meetings addressed by John Foster showed that this problem of interests had to be talked through and taken seriously. There could not be (should not be?) an automatic presumption that citizens in insecure employment positions should privilege those who work for the community. So leadership takes place in a pluralistic set of relations. Concepts of leadership that assume a universal interest in this context are false. After all, democratic society became popular because it demonstrated that it was good at handling conflict and disagreement, not because there was a single set of interests in society.

In the Jobcentre Plus case the leader had to handle trade union resistance to the changes. It could be seen as about a change of public service culture. Trade union activists at Jobcentre Plus saw removal of the screened environment in the new integrated offices as a health and safety issue. For the managerial leadership the safety issue had to be considered alongside the customer service issue. This case is a perfect illustration of the way the new welfare state is not only about moving away from 'passive' support to 'active' support but also about putting the public first and providing good service. It appeared that this agenda could only be advanced by a leadership prepared to face up to the need to change the organisation's culture and confront conflict.

Lesson Three: leaders know the detail

We have identified attention to detail as an important attribute of public services leadership. The trouble with oversimplified pictures of visionary leadership is that it appears that all is needed is for the leader to communicate the 'big picture' and then empowered managers and employees are inspired to take action. Our rejection of this is informed by the example of Wendy Thomson at Newham Council. But, as we have already noted, this is consistent with conclusions reported by Borins (1998) based on his analysis of turnaround cases in the public sector.

Lesson Four: leaders have to be resilient

The idea of visionary leadership suggests leaders inspire followers. Occasionally writers suggest that leaders energise their followers and that this energy is important for the change process. But we have found that leaders have to have energy and resilience to cope with resistance and even personal attacks that arise because of the disruption caused by change.

Lesson Five: 'standalone is not the only way'

When considering both the literature and practice around public service leadership it is necessary to acknowledge the importance of exhibiting a capacity for creativity and innovation. This can, as we have seen, be construed in a number of ways, but primarily can be said to break down across two thematic streams:

- Using internal resources and structures differently
- Exploiting the potential for partnership with other organisations, be they in the public service, not for profit or commercial sectors.

The first of these streams is an approach that can be seen by almost every senior-level leader within the first year of their taking up post. Reviewing internal operations and associated organisational design can be said to be a recognised part of the new leader's 'toolkit'. Some will be more successful at it than others, particularly in respect of articulating the requirement for review and change to a wider stakeholder group. Bennis argues that such activity represents the commencement of the innovation cycle in an individual's engagement with an organisation:

> 'He does things other people haven't done or don't do. He does things in advance of other people. He makes new things. He makes old things new. Having learned from the past, he lives in the present, with one eye on the future. And each leader puts it all together in a different way . . .. They must be intuitive, conceptual, synthesising and artistic.'
>
> (Bennis 1959: 143)

If we reflect on the example of Centrelink that we explored in Chapter 3, we can see that this model of leadership marries closely with the approach adopted by Sue Vardon when appointed as Chief Executive. Her approach could certainly be described as both 'intuitive and conceptual' – taking on board the challenges of an organisation created from the merging of disparate parts of other 'service lines'. The questions that she required the organisation to ask of itself and of its entire rationale for existing, were based around what was hitherto an often forgotten concept, that of placing the service user at the heart of service design issues. The creativity and capacity for internal service innovation that flowed from this initial approach represent one of the best 'lessons' in organisational leadership that we can observe internationally today. And interestingly, this approach served as a platform, to create an organisation which had the confidence and maturity, to then look externally to partner with other organisations both within and without the public service environment to both develop and enhance the scale and scope of offerings to clients.

Taking forward this theme of developing organisational capacity through partnership, we do then need to consider the public service leader as being comfortable with contracting relationships with other suppliers. Now of course, for over two decades we have seen public services globally engage in a variety of 'contracting out' arrangements whereby third parties are contracted to deliver services on behalf of the public service authority. Leaders within this context have been largely concerned with the achievement of best value and of monitoring performance levels against agreed standards. However, such approaches have not, in the main, been marked out by any sense of innovation permeating what largely remain rather traditionally structured public service structures. Here the emphasis is upon the contractual arrangement rather than the potential benefits of partnership. Leadbetter identifies this as a major political and policy challenge and argues that:

> 'Public sector organizations are seen as highly change resistant and as poor at innovation. They could be revitalized by a new breed of managers such as "turnaround" headmasters in failing schools who seek to secure more value from the public assets that they are stewards of . . .. There is a need for more entrepreneurial and creative orientation which could create a greater range of innovative public services . . . empowering of public sector innovators and "social entrepreneurs" is difficult as traditional vertically organized accountability mechanisms stress the virtues of predictability and standardization.'
>
> (McLaughlin *et al.* 2002: 349)

Challenging 'predictability and standardization' could stand as fitting epitaphs for the impact of David Henshaw's leadership that was discussed in Chapter 7. In his own words he sets out a vision of public service which has no problems in 'passing the baton' to other providers when doing so, and clearly represents the most creative opportunity for gaining a better service experience for the citizen. His leadership *courage* in constructing the rationale for Liverpool Direct, the joint venture organisation with BT, serves as an example of genuine creativity. The motivation for its creation was not unique – the need to modernise technology infrastructures in order to support service redesign and development – the organisational setting was particularly dire. Many labelled Liverpool as an organisation quite beyond hope. However, due to leadership vision, and an organisational context which was so poor that the potential for real innovation could not be sensibly challenged by internal stakeholders, a model of partnership and governance developed which remains an example from which most public service structures can learn useful lessons.

Perhaps the strongest message to emerge from the example of Liverpool Direct, is that of the importance of public service leaders having both the vision and confidence to move from a relationship of *client* and *contractor*, to that of *partner* in a change agenda. Such a shift of mind-set is one which for many public service leaders represents a major stepping outside of comfort zones established and reinforced over the decades of the 1980s and 1990s. Even leaders who have proved themselves adept at developing the capacity to innovate and be creative internally, can find the leap of faith involved in working with external parties as partners, to be too great to contemplate.

However, the natural progression of the theme of NPM and our allied assertion that a new public service leadership paradigm must sit alongside it, suggests that new relationships and mechanisms for working outside traditional boundaries represent the natural progression of the position we currently find ourselves in. The journey which began in the 1990s which saw an encouragement of *blurring* of service lines between strands of public service offering, has gathered pace and we now find ourselves facing a future where the demarcation lines between what is provided by the public sector directly, and what is not, become increasingly blurred also. Leadership within the public service arena will increasingly demand that those in the most senior positions are able to demonstrate a capacity to invite and encourage an environment of multi-provider working. Such leaders must also be capable of engendering the confidence of other types of organisation, that they have the capacity and willingness to work as partners over time, and the insight and imagination to ensure that corporate governance prioritises opportunities for learning and development. Clearly the lesson learned here, is that it is unlikely to be desirable, or indeed possible, to aspire to be a senior public service leader, without demonstrating a capacity and enthusiasm for grasping all the many challenges of social entrepreneurship.

Lesson Six: 'Eat and drink less, and laugh more: don't think you have to be unpleasant to be strong!' (Parker 1989: 110)

Being a successful leader, as we have discussed throughout this book, almost without exception, requires that the individual must possess the capability to *adapt* to increasingly fluid and challenging operating environments. Our concept of adaptive leadership represents an overarching theme within the wider leadership context. However, in terms of the specific learning that we would take from it here, it can be said to refer to many personal qualities, most of which are intuitively held, and which many argue cannot be taught. All of the leaders we have discussed and critiqued within this text, share a common theme of success attained within challenging public service environments. Yet, as a group of people, they are marked out by the diversity of the personality traits that they exhibit – however simplistic it may appear, it is important to record, that just as all human beings are unique, so too are those who we may otherwise 'label' under the generic term leader.

The quotation from Peter Parker used at the outset of this lesson reflects the humour with which this successful leader was able to draw upon his own experiential learning. Whilst undoubtedly his own particular recipe for leadership might be characterised as rather more from the operational than the conceptual perspective, embedded within soundbites such as 'if you are in a hanging mood, hang people like pictures – in the best light', there is encapsulated a leadership philosophy which is meaningful and important within the contexts with which we are concerned (Parker 1989: 110). Undoubtedly the leaders we have considered within this text are all different people – yet, if one considers the areas of commonality, they coalesce around the set of behaviours that the leader exhibits when dealing with individuals, groups and the whole organisation. Demonstrating respect for others and resilience in communicating new challenges, as well as being marked out by the integrity with which they undertake a change agenda, would appear to sum up the leadership behaviours that we have observed in our research for this book. These points emerged in Chapter 2 as well as in our case studies.

As more and more leadership academies are established by governments, anxious to develop and enhance the leadership capacity within their public services, we need to question the extent to which behaviours can be taught. Our conclusions, based upon what we have observed, is that the greatest opportunities for learning and development, whether within discrete academies, or development programmes, actually arise from having the opportunity to interact with, and learn from, other good exemplars of successful leadership behaviours. Bennis has an interesting and useful perspective on how one becomes a successful leader:

'Learning to lead, is on one level, learning to manage change. As we have seen, a leader imposes (in the most positive sense of the word) his philosophy on the organization, creating or re-creating its culture. The organization then acts on that philosophy, carries out a mission, and the culture takes on a life of its own, becoming more cause than effect. But unless the leader continues to evolve, to adapt and adjust to external change, the organization will sooner or later stall.

In other words, one of the leader's principal gifts is his ability to use his experiences to grow in office . . ... Leaders learn by leading, and they learn the best by leading in the face of obstacles. As weather shapes mountains, so problems make leaders . . ... Today there are risks in being at the head of the pack. You can get shot in the back. People try to trip you. People want you to fail. And at some point or another, every leader falls off his pedestal. They are either pulled down, shot down, or they do something dumb, or they just wear out.'

(Bennis 1989: 143–7)

Bennis's point of conclusion is an important aspect of this lesson in leadership – that being that whilst leaders must exhibit courage, energy, resilience and even good humour, they are, just as their political counterparts most assuredly are, marked by a time span of value and usefulness. To stay beyond the point at which the leader and the led are enjoying mutual confidence in one another, and sharing a willingness and energy to sustain change, is to invite the potential to be remembered for the end of the journey, rather than for the successes achieved along the way. Strong and effective leaders not only exemplify excellence in operating in the present and the future, they shape organisations that can sustain and benefit from a future without them.

Lesson Seven: leadership is all about change

At the risk of stating the obvious, the lessons that have preceded build a picture where the clearest discernible pattern of behaviour in analysing successful public service leaders, is one which sees the drive for change on an ongoing basis as being a key determinant of success. Change stemming from ideological shifts can lead us to map a trajectory that might be said to have begun with excellence being seen to stem from bureaucratic structures; through the construction of a Welfare State model, that moved the scale of the bureaucratic model into the realms of a scope and scale that many developed nations have struggled to sustain. The response to this in the 1980s and early 1990s was the development of liberal capitalism, which theoretically sought to diminish the role of the state, without always following through on this in the development and deployment of policy. To the point where we find ourselves now, where the state once more seeks to reinvent its role, serving and responding to citizens in ways which are held to be customer-facing and -engaging. Ferlie, the early architect of the NPM concept, considers that the journey is a sustainable one:

> '. . . the organization and management of . . . public services has undergone an archetype shift from a previously dominant public administration archetype to a novel NPM archetype. This shift is a successful reorientation and is far more deep-rooted than the usual managerial fad or fashion.'
>
> (McLaughlin *et al.* 2002: 352)

What we can take from this 'pen portrait' analysis of the political trajectory, is that the change agenda at almost every change has been enormous in policy terms. For public service leaders, the challenge in responding to this evolution of public policy directions, has been that the most successful have learned a leadership style which ensures that they create organisations which are future-facing.

Leading public service organisations with radar focused on the present and the future has been one of the key revolutions that we can cite, in the development of a credible perspective on new public service leadership. Whilst the leaders of public services for many generations were schooled to essentially *manage* a reasonably constant operating environment; those who have come to prominence globally in the last decade, have been marked out by their ability to embrace the opportunities of emergent political perspectives, and to interpret them successfully within new models of public service. Change management for those leaders in this group, has been rather more about creating within public service organisations a capacity to embrace and sustain change, than about managing a linear process. Indeed, it is very unlikely that any change attempted in the public services has been, or will be, perfect from the point of the leader's actions. However, the learning we can take from each attempt to make public services reform happen is actually very important.

Tushman, whose analysis of organisational renewal we discussed in Chapter 4, believes that all organisations, regardless of their sector, go through a period of transition from being change enabled, through to having the capacity to renew. Most organisations probably occupy various stages of the transition phase. Building a capacity for change, we would argue, is possibly the single most important lesson that can be taken from this analysis. Tushman argues that it is at this phase that the role of leadership is at its most crucial – again, a view with which we would concur.

We are fortunate in the cases that we have cited within this work, to have had access to a number of leaders whose behaviour and achievements closely align to this concept of visionary leadership. Perhaps the final point that Tushman makes, around the creation of a 'personal bond' between the leader and the organisation, is the most important determinant of success that our research has identified when considering the readiness or otherwise of organisations to take on innovation and change agendas. To take the example of David Henshaw at Liverpool City Council, the sense that he and the organisation are inextricably entwined, permeates almost every interaction with those working within the council. Given both the external perceptions and internal realities of this organisation, to have such a strong and indeed visionary leadership figure at the forefront of all change activities, was arguably the only way to begin an agenda of change. However, as we discussed in relation to lesson six, most leadership roles are characterised by a timeframe which can only be successful for as long as the leader and the led are both motivated and energised by the same agenda. Visionary leaders are certainly essential at the transition phase in any public service change programme – however, it is absolutely critical to acknowledge that leadership style and/or the leader themselves, may not actually be the most appropriate choice to lead the organisation towards its next stage of development.

Lesson Eight: Leaders develop an organisational capability to *renew* rather than change in isolation

Some organisations develop a capacity to continually evolve and renew themselves in a manner which is altogether more seamless and fluid than the processes most often associated with a change agenda. Reaching such a position is something that can only be achieved over time and requires the building of both confidence and leadership capacity across the whole organisation. Within a public service environment the challenges associated with attainment of such a position are complicated by the relative instability of the operating environment and the allied complexity associated with having to operate within a politically driven policy and strategy environment.

Whilst acknowledging the difficulties associated with the particular challenges of operating in the public services sector, one should not dismiss the aspiration to develop organisations which are capable of renewing their mission, focus, and service offering as part of 'normal business' as opposed to change activity. It is reasonable to posit a view that all top-level leaders should aspire to create organisations that are capable of renewal.

Once again the overarching theme emerging here relates to the concept of an *adaptive* approach to leadership as being an essential characteristic of an effective approach to leadership. Certainly in respect of moving towards the development of a renewal-focused organisation, the capacity for the most senior leaders to demonstrate adaptive characteristics would appear to be absolutely critical in moving beyond the first stages of change management. As we have discussed, the realities of the operating environment are such that without a capacity to adapt and to communicate such adjustments in direction successfully, the likelihood of enjoying the sustained benefits of leadership are minimal. The lesson to be learned around renewal is that it should feature prominently on the radar of any senior-level leader, as an aspiration to work towards. The emphasis that it places upon leveraging the organisational capacity to subsume change within a normal working agenda, is one which can only be built over time. The key requirement to achieve this organisational mind-set is that of confidence permeating the organisation and exhibited across all the many leadership roles that can be found within public service organisations.

Organisational renewal can be viewed as an abstract concept, so removed can it appear from the realities of seeking to lead and manage organisations in complex and challenging environments. However, if leadership is itself to mature as a key determinant of public service success, then it must be predicated upon a belief that leadership is about a rather longer journey than that represented by an aspiration to lead change. Without a focus upon a renewal agenda, then it is possible to argue that both leadership and change management activities remain characterised by their application and relevance at only a 'moment in time'. Focusing upon engendering a capacity to renew, is about delivering a sustainable capacity to deliver appropriate public services as a matter of course.

Lesson Nine: walking a tightrope – leadership within NPM

Leadership as both a concept, and an individual and organisational aspiration, has gained such prominence within recent years, that one might be forgiven for believing that this is the key determinant of success. Whilst certainly we feel that in the case studies and examples referred to in this text, the prominent and even pivotal role played by effective leadership, has been clearly established, we must acknowledge also, that leadership in isolation is unlikely to bring about successful or sustainable organisational change and development. It is possible to argue that the spotlight on leadership as the single most important ingredient in attaining increased levels of success, is to be expected, because in simple 'visibility' rankings, it is the factor which most stakeholders will feel they have some awareness of.

The reality is that the public service reform agenda that has been driven globally by NPM, has little place within its philosophical or operating lexicon, for the term 'failure'. Whilst, of course, it is important to acknowledge that in any other sector, failure that has detrimental impact on bottom-line performance, will not be tolerated for long, the public service environment does throw up some leadership challenges and stresses which are uniquely its own. The environment, within which public service leaders typically have to operate, is increasingly characterised by a dominance of performance measurement and allied indicators. Within a leadership context these can be viewed in two main ways; the first is that such measures actually serve as proxies for effective service leadership and allied strategic development. Within this model, it could be argued that NPM has set forth a view that leadership within the public service environment is somehow a proposition that is fatally undermined by the bureaucratic and change-resistant cultures that it seeks to replace, and that therefore a prescriptive and centralised response is required.

However, emerging from our case material and interpretation of the wider leadership debate, we feel more inclined to suggest that the drivers of NPM, namely performance enhancement and measurement, have made possible a more viable and visible style of leadership, which we have referred to as New Public Service Leadership. Within this interpretation, innovative and change-orientated approaches to leadership have actually been enabled by the establishment of a political will, for public services to be reformed in ways which are meaningful to the citizen as end user. The use of performance metrics, often it must be said in quantities whose value must be questioned, have served to set out a clear road map for sustained change. Successful leaders operating in such environments typically harness the many stresses and reporting requirements of targets and performance indicators, and use them to effectively challenge ingrained and change-resistant behaviours.

Leaders in this environment must perform a delicate balancing act, which ensures conformance with externally set targets, whilst at the same time creating organisations which can meet and exceed such targets without ultimately being aware that they are doing so. Creating and sustaining innovative and performance-focused public services is the ultimate challenge in public service leadership that is evident internationally today. The performance- and conformance-orientated environments that are being increasingly the norm, are challenging and unforgiving environments in which to work. Which perhaps leads us to conclude that the logical consequence of lessons one to eight, is that lesson nine must be, that not all public service managers have the leadership qualities, and in particular the resilience, to take on the challenges of being at the forefront of public service leadership. The reality is that very few have the personal and organisational skills and instincts to operate as successful leaders. Taken as a whole, there is much that those with an interest in new public service leadership can take from Mark Twain's observation that:

'Two things seemed pretty apparent to me. One was, that in order to be a Mississippi River pilot a man had got to learn more than any one man ought to be allowed to know; and the other was, that he must learn it all over again in a different way every twenty-four hours.'

(Twain 2000: 63)

CONCLUSION

The overall theme of this final chapter is that leadership is about change, but not just change in the abstract. From the 1940s to the end of the 1960s was the heyday of the old welfare state society. Between 1979 and 1997, the British state attempted to restore a society based on liberal capitalism. This failed to happen and in the 21st century a process of reconstruction began not only of the welfare services but also of the relationship between the public services and the public being served.

Leadership is caught up in the reconstruction task. During the preceding period – Thatcherism – the issue was to manage the welfare state efficiently (while hoping to reduce it) for as long as it continued to exist – not to change it and modernise it. Perhaps the evidence of Thatcherism was that the welfare state could not be simply abolished. Perhaps society finds the welfare state both a burden on business and taxpayers but also indispensable. Nothing we have said should be taken as assuming that it will be easy to redesign the welfare state.

We would like to conclude this book with the idea that managerial leaders in the new public services offer 'hope' not salvation. Hope is different from both the certainty that elite models of leadership seem to imply and the cynicism that imbues the discourse perspective. Leadership that offers hope might be seen as synthesis of the other two states. Because it is only hope and not certainty that can be offered, we would say it should also morally be democratic. If a leader cannot claim certainty, then the options and consequences need a discussion of options and consequences that is inclusive.

BIBLIOGRAPHY

Alban-Metcalfe, R. and Alimo-Metcalfe, B. (2000) 'The Transformational Leadership Questionnaire (TLQ-LGV): a Convergent and Discriminant Validation Study', *Leadership & Organization Development Journal*, 21(6): 280–96.

Alimo-Metcalfe, B. (2003) 'Stamp of Greatness', *Health Service Journal*, 26 June 2003, 28–32.

Alimo-Metcalfe, B. and Alban-Metcalfe, R.J. (2001) 'The development of a new Transformational Leadership Questionnaire', *Journal of Occupational and Organizational Psychology*, 74: 1–27.

Alimo-Metcalfe, B. and Alban-Metcalfe, J. (2002) 'The Great and the Good', *People Management*, 8(1): 32–4.

Alimo-Metcalfe, B. and Alban-Metcalfe, J. (2003) 'Under the Influence', *People Management*, 16 March: 32–5.

Alimo-Metcalfe, B. and Lawler, J. (2001) 'Leadership Development in UK Companies at the Beginning of the Twenty-first Century: Lessons for the NHS?' *Journal of Management in Medicine*, 15(5): 387–404.

Audit Commission (2002) *Liverpool City Council: Corporate Assessment*. London: Audit Commission.

Audit Commission (2003) *Targets in the Public Sector*. London: Audit Commission.

Barnard C. I. (1938) *The Functions of the Executive*. Cambridge, MA: Harvard University Press.

Bass, B. M. (1985) *Leadership and Performance Beyond Expectations*. New York: Free Press.

Bass, B. M. and Avolio, B. J. (1990) 'Training and development of transformational leadership for individual, team and organizational development,' in: R. W. Woodman and W. A. Passmore (eds) *Research in Organizational Change and Development*. Greenwich, CT: JAI Press.

Bennis, W. (1959) 'Leadership Theory and Administrative Behavior: the Problem of Authority', *Administrative Science Quarterly*, 4(3): 259–301.

Bennis, W. (2000) *Old Dogs, New Tricks*. London: Kogan Page.

Bennis, W. (2002) 'A Farewell to the Old Leadership', in *Leadership and Management in the Information Age*. Abu Dhabi: The Emirates Center for Strategic Studies and Research.

Bennis, W. and Nanus, B. (1985) *Leaders: The Strategies for Taking Charge*. New York: Harper & Row.

Berman, E. and Wang, X. (2000) 'Performance Measurement in US Counties: Capacity for Reform', *Public Administration Review*, September/October, 60(5): 409–20.

Beveridge Report (1942) *Social Insurance and Allied Services*. Cmd 6404, 6405. London: HMSO.

Beveridge, W. H. (1944) *Full Employment in a Free Society*. London: Allen & Unwin.

Bichard, M. (2000) 'Creativity, Leadership and Change', *Public Money and Management*, April–June: 41–6.

Boehnke, K. Bontis, N., Distefano, J. J. and Distefano, A.C. (2003) 'Transformational Leadership: an Examination of Cross-national Differences and Similarities', *Leadership & Organisation Development*, 24(1): 5–15.

Borins, S. (1998) *Innovating with Integrity: How Local Heroes Are Transforming American Government*. Washington: Georgetown University Press.

Bryman, A. (1992) *Charisma and Leadership in Organizations*. London: Sage.

Buchanan, D. and Badham, R. (1999) *Power, Politics and Organizational Change*. London: Sage Publications.

Cabinet Office (2001) *Open All Hours – a Report on Extended Service Hours*. London: Cabinet Office Modernising Public Services Report.

CEML (no date) *Excellent Managers and Leaders: Meeting the Need*. London: the Council for Excellence in Management and Leadership.

Charlesworth, K., Cook, P. and Crozier, G. (2003) *Leading Change in the Public Sector: Making the Difference*. London: Chartered Management Institute.

Clarke, J., Cochrane, A. and McLaughlin, E. (1994) 'Introduction: Why Management Matters', in J. Clarke, A. Cochrane and E. McLaughlin (eds) *Managing Social Policy*. London: Sage Publications.

Clarke, J., Gewirtz, S. and McLaughlin, E. (2000) *New Managerialism, New Welfare?* London: Sage Publications.

Cole, G. D. H. (1947) *The Intelligent Man's Guide to the Post-War World*. London: Victor Gollancz.

Cole, G. D. H. and Postgate, R. (1949) *The Common People: 1746–1946*. London: Methuen.

Collins, J. (2001) 'Level 5 Leadership', *Harvard Business Review*, 79(1): 66–76.

Corrigan, P. and Joyce, P. (1997) 'Reconstructing Public Management: A New Responsibility for the Public' and 'A Case Study of Local Government', *International Journal of Public Sector Management*, 10(6): 417–32.

Crainer, S. (ed.) (1996) *Leaders on Leadership.* Corby: Institute of Management.

Department for Education and Skills and Department of Trade and Industry (2002) *Managers and Leaders: Raising our Game.* London: Department for Education and Skills.

Deutsch, K. W. (1966) *The Nerves of Government: Models of Political Communication and Control.* New York: Free Press.

Doh, J. P. (2003) 'Can Leadership Be Taught? Perspectives from Management Educators', *Academy of Management Learning and Education*, 2(1): 54–67.

Donnelly, L. (2003) 'Kennedy Sparks CHAI Row', *Health Service Journal*, 5 June: 7.

Dovey, K. (2002) 'Leadership Development in a South African Health Service', *International Journal of Public Sector Management*, 15(7): 520–33.

Duncan, W. J., Ginter, P. M. and Swayne, L. E. (1995) *Strategic Management of Health Care Organizations.* Oxford: Blackwell.

Elcock, H. (2001) *Political Leadership.* Cheltenham: Edward Elgar.

Faerman, S. R., Quinn, R. E. and Thompson, M. P. (1987) 'Bridging Management Practice and Theory: New York State's Public Service Training Program', *Public Administration Review*, July/August, 47(4): 310–19.

Fenlon, M. (2002) 'The Public Spirit', *Financial Times*, 22 November: 4–5.

Ferlie, E. (2000) The Sustainability of the New Public Management in the UK, Symposium Paper for the Annual Conference of the American Academy of Management, Toronto, August 2000.

Ferlie, E., Ashburner, L., Fitzgerald, L. and Pettigrew, A. (1996) *The New Public Management.* Oxford: Oxford University Press.

Follett, M. P. (1941) *Dynamic Administration: The Collected Papers of Mary Parker Follett.* Bath: Management Publications Trust.

Friedman, B. (1998) *Delivering on the Promise: How to Attract, Manage and Return Human Capital.* New York: Free Press.

Frost-Kumpf, L., Wechsler, B., Ishiyama, H. J. and Backoff, R. W. (1993) 'Strategic Action and Transformational Change: The Ohio Department of Mental Health', in B. Bozeman (ed.) *Public Management: The State of the Art.* San Francisco: Jossey-Bass.

Gabris, G. T., Grenell, K., Ihrke, D. and Kaatz, J. (1999) 'Managerial Innovation as affected by Administrative Leadership and Policy Boards', *Public Administration Quarterly*, 23(2): 223–50.

Gabris, G., Golembiewski, R. and Ihrke, D. (2000) 'Leadership Credibility, Board Relations, and Administrative Innovation at the Local Government Level', *Journal of Public Administration Research and Theory*, 11(1): 89–108.

Gellis, Z. D. (2001) 'Social Work Perceptions of Transformational and Transactional Leadership in Health Care', *Social Work Research*, 25(1): 17–25.

Giddens, A. (1998) *The Third Way: the Renewal of Social Democracy.* London: Polity Press.

Giuliani, R. (2002) 'Giuliani on Restoring Accountability to City Government', *PwC Journal*, Summer.

Goffee, R. and Jones, G. (2002) 'The Traits of Good Leadership', *Financial Times*, 1 November: 4–5.

Hamel, G. (2002) *Leading the Revolution*. Boston, MA: Harvard Business School Press.

Hamel, G. and Prahalad, C. K. (1994) *Competing for the Future*. Boston, MA: Harvard Business School Press.

Handy, C. (1994) *The Empty Raincoat*. London: Arrow.

Heifetz, R. A. and Linsky, M. (2002) *Leadership on the Line*. Boston, MA: Harvard Business School Press.

Heifetz, R. and Laurie, D. (1997) 'The Work of Leadership', *Harvard Business Review*, January–February: 187–97.

Herb, E. Leslie, K. and Price, C. (2001) 'Teamwork at the Top', The McKinsey Quarterly, 2. http://www.mckinseyquarterly.com/article_page.asp?ar51022&L2518&L =32 (downloaded 24 July 2002).

Heymann, P. B. (1987) *The Politics of Public Management*. New Haven, CT and London: Yale University Press.

Hood, C. (1991) 'A New Public Management for All Seasons?', *Public Administration* 69(1): 3–19.

Hooijberg, R. and Choi, J. (2001) 'The Impact of Organizational Characteristics on Leadership Effectiveness Models: an Examination of Leadership in a Private and a Public Sector Organization', *Administration and Society*, 33(4): 403–31.

Javidan, M. and Waldman, D. A. (2003) 'Exploring Charismatic Leadership in the Public Sector: Measurement and Consequences', *Public Administration Review*, 63(2): 229–242.

Joyce, P. (1999) *Strategic Management for the Public Services*. Buckingham: Open University Press.

Joyce, P. (2000) *Strategy in the Public Sector: A Guide to Effective Change Management*. Chichester: Wiley.

Kanter, R. M. (1997) *On the Frontiers of Management*. Boston, MA: Harvard Business Review Publishing.

Kellerman, B. and Webster, S. W. (2001) 'The Recent Literature on Public Leadership Reviewed and Considered', *The Leadership Quarterly*, 12: 485–514.

Kilfoyle, P. and Parker, I. (2000) *Left behind: Issues from Labour's Heartland*. London: Politico.

Kim, W. and Mauborgne, R. (2003) 'Fair Process: Managing in the Knowledge Economy', *Harvard Business Review*, January.

Kim, W., Maugborne, R. and Van der Heyden, L. (2002) 'General Failings', *Financial Times*, 6 December: 4–5.

Kotter, J. (1990) 'What Leaders Really Do', *Harvard Business Review*, May–June.

Kouzes, J. and Posner, B. (1990) 'The Credibility Factor: What Followers Expect from their Leaders', *Management Review*, (79)1: 29–33.

Le Brasseur, R., Whissell, R. and Ojha, A. (2002) 'Organisational Learning, Transformational Leadership and Implementation of Continuous Quality Improvement in Canadian Hospitals', *Australian Journal of Management*, 27(2): 141–62.

Liverpool City Council (2003) *Review of Service Improvement.* Liverpool: Liverpool City Council.

Liverpool Direct Ltd (2003) *Liverpool Direct Ltd, A Review of Services.* Liverpool: Liverpool Direct Ltd.

Local Government Ombudsman (2001) Report on an Investigation into Complaint No. 99/A/4226 against the London Borough of Southwark, 21 Queen Anne's Gate, London SW1H 9BU.

Loffler, E. and Klages, H. (1995) 'Administrative Modernization in Germany – a Big Qualitative Jump in Small Steps', *International Review of Administrative Sciences*, 61: 373–83.

MacKenzie, N. and Mackenzie, J. (1977) *The First Fabians.* London: Quartet.

McLaughlin, K., Osborne, S. and Ferlie, E. (eds) (2002) *New Public Management, Current Trends and Future Prospects.* London: Routledge.

Milner, E. (2002) *Delivering the Vision: Public Services for the Information Society and the Knowledge Economy.* London: Routledge.

Mintzberg, H. (1995) 'Beyond Configuration: Forces and Forms in Effective Organizations', in H. Mintzberg, J. B. Quinn, and S. Ghoshal (eds), *The Strategy Process.* London: Prentice Hall.

Moore, M. (1995) *Creating Public Value: Strategic Management in Government.* London: Harvard University Press.

Newman, J. and Clarke, J. (1994) 'Going about Our Business? The Managerialization of Public Services', in J. Clarke, A. Cochrane, and E. McLaughlin (eds) *Managing Social Policy.* London: Sage.

NHS Modernisation Agency (2003) *Leading Change in the Modern NHS.* Leicester: NHS Modernisation Agency.

O'Brien, G. (2002) 'Participation as the Key to Successful Change', *Leadership and Organization Development Journal*, 23(8): 442–55.

OECD (Organisation for Economic Co-operation and Development) (1995) *Governance in Transition: Public Management Reforms in OECD Countries.* Paris: OECD.

Osborne, D., and Gaebler, T. (1992) *Reinventing Government: How the Entrepreneurial Spirit is Transforming the Public Sector.* Reading, MA: Addison-Wesley.

Owen, D. (1965) *English Philanthropy 1660–1960.* Boston: Bellknapp Press.

Parker, P. (1989) *For Starters.* London: Jonathan Cape.

Parry, K. W. (1999) 'Enhancing Adaptability: Leadership Strategies to Accommodate Change in Local Government Settings', *Journal of Organizational Change Management*, 12(2): 134–56.

Performance and Innovation Unit (2001) *Strengthening Leadership in the Public Sector.*

Peters, T. and Waterman, R. (1982) *In Search of Excellence*. New York: HarperCollins.

Pettigrew, A. (2001) 'What Makes Good Leadership?', *Interchange News*, London: NHS Confederation

Pettigrew, A. and Whipp, R. (1993) *Managing Change for Competitive Success*. Oxford: Blackwell.

Pettigrew, A., Ferlie, E. and McKee, L. (1992) *Shaping Strategic Change*. London: Sage.

Pollitt, C. (1993) *The New Managerialism and the Public Services*. Oxford: Basil Blackwell.

Pollitt, C., Birchall, J. and Putnam, K. (1998) *Decentralising Public Service Management*. London: Macmillan.

Schacter, H. (1994) Revolution from within. *Canadian Business*, 67: 31–47.

Senge, P. (1999) *The Dance of Change*. London: Nicholas Brealey.

Senge, P. M., Kleiner, A., Roberts, C., Ross, R. B. and Smith, B. J. (1994) *The Fifth Discipline Fieldbook: Strategies and Tools for Building a Learning Organization*. London: Doubleday.

Tushman, M. and O'Reilly, C. (2002) *Winning through Innovation: a Practical Guide to Leading Organizational Change and Renewal*. Boston, MA: Harvard Business School Press.

Twain, M. (2000) *Life on the Mississippi*. London: Dover Books.

Walsh, K. (1995) *Public Services and Market Mechanisms*. London: Macmillan.

Webber, A. (1986) 'The Statesman as CEO: James Callaghan', *Harvard Business Review*, November–December: 108–12.

Webber, A. (1987) 'The Statesman as CEO: Gerald Ford', *Harvard Business Review*, September–October: 76–80.

Weber, M. (1947) *The Theory of Social and Economic Organization*. London: The Free Press.

Weber, M. (1970) *From Max Weber: Essays in Sociology*, edited by H. H. Gerth and C. Wright Mills. London: Routledge & Kegan Paul.

Zaleznik, A. (1977) 'Managers and Leaders: Are They Different?', *Harvard Business Review:* May–June: 23–7.

INDEX